Deprescribing in Psychiatry

Deprescribing in Psychiatry

SWAPNIL GUPTA, MBBS, MD
REBECCA MILLER, PHD
JOHN D. CAHILL, BMBS, PHD
Yale University School of Medicine
Department of Psychiatry
New Haven, Connecticut

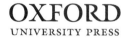
OXFORD
UNIVERSITY PRESS

OXFORD
UNIVERSITY PRESS

Oxford University Press is a department of the University of Oxford. It furthers the University's objective of excellence in research, scholarship, and education by publishing worldwide. Oxford is a registered trade mark of Oxford University Press in the UK and certain other countries.

Published in the United States of America by Oxford University Press
198 Madison Avenue, New York, NY 10016, United States of America.

© Oxford University Press 2019

Library of Congress Cataloging-in-Publication Data
Names: Gupta, Swapnil, author. | Miller, Rebecca, 1974– author. | Cahill, John (John D.), author.
Title: Deprescribing in psychiatry / Swapnil Gupta, Rebecca Miller, John Cahill.
Description: New York, NY : Oxford University Press, [2019] |
Includes bibliographical references.
Identifiers: LCCN 2019012605| ISBN 9780190654818 (pbk.) |
ISBN 9780190654825 (UPDF) | ISBN 9780190654832 (ePub) |
Subjects: | MESH: Mental Disorders—drug therapy | Deprescriptions |
Psychotropic Drugs—adverse effects | Inappropriate
Prescribing—prevention & control | Mental Health Recovery
Classification: LCC RC483 | NLM WM 402 | DDC 616.89/18—dc23
LC record available at https://lccn.loc.gov/2019012605

3 5 7 9 8 6 4 2

Printed by Marquis, Canada

To Gyan, SSJ, and Rajo. SG
To JR — thank you for sharing the decision with me. RM
To V (and all others with the wisdom and courage to have more questions than answers). JC

Contents

Preface

Many of us also know what it means to be buried under an avalanche of psychiatric drugs. We know what it means to have the treatment be worse than the disorder. We know what it means to be in a chemical tomb, where we feel so drugged we are neither alive nor dead; when we are so drugged that our bodies are stiff and slow and lifeless; when our faces become expressionless masks; when our eyes stop dancing and, instead, glaze over into a petrified stare; when our passion is neutered under powerful pharmaceuticals; and when we are, quite literally, disappeared within a chemical coma.

—Deegan (2004)

This provocative and disturbing description of one person's experience of taking an excess of psychiatric meds is, unfortunately, not a unique experience. With the growth of pharmaceutical approaches to treating psychological distress and psychiatric symptoms, psychiatric prescribers are more equipped to add, rather than take away. Without sounding overly ambitious, this book aims to take a step toward rebalancing the scales by promoting the innovation, implementation and study of *rational deprescribing as an intervention for psychiatry*. We, the authors, do not approach the topic lightly, having seen the great benefits of awakening a person's spirit when medications address signs and symptoms appropriately and allow a person to regain or establish a life they love. We do not profess to have the singular algorithm for determining who needs what medication and when (i.e., who would benefit from what medication at what dose and for what length of time). We do not presume that the individual prescriber reading this should necessarily be prescribing fewer medications, nor do we consider deprescribing a panacea. Furthermore, deprescribing should not be regarded as a movement or a fad.

Instead, our more modest proposal is to offer a pragmatic starting point; and to stimulate open conversation among patient, prescriber, the clinical team, and friends and family in order to support the option of decreasing or stopping psychiatric medications through a process of shared decision-making: the intervention of *deprescribing*. While Deegan's quoted description may seem extreme, it is not an uncommon experience, particularly for those with psychotic disorders. Many of our own patients and many patients across the country are prescribed multiple psychotropic medications, especially during a hospital stay, with varying degrees of follow-up evaluation of their purpose and ongoing necessity. Polypharmacy is prevalent, carrying numerous often underconsidered risks.

This book and we the authors are not "anti-psychiatry". In fact we view deprescribing as a tool with which psychiatry might remain most relevant and effective moving into the future. Two of us are practicing psychiatrists (SG, JC) who make ample use of medications in their practice, and the other is a practicing psychologist (RM), all working in an active urban community mental health setting. Instead we might consider ourselves "anti-irrational prescribing". To put it in a more strengths-based frame, we consider ourselves interested in promoting a person's best life by using the tools to support that objective in the most reasonable way, tools that include medications and psychotherapy along with a whole host of others. At the same time, we look to collaborating and leaving appropriate room for individual testing to see if medications are useful tools for the person in this pursuit, and if so, which and how much. It comes from a place of humility rather than hubris that we imagine this book as in its first edition. Our hope is that a seed has been planted and that, with time, the field's experience and evidence base will grow—and so too will this volume. Part 1 reflects context, selected background and rationale that drives this work for us. Part 2 proposes a starting point for the development of deprescribing clinical guidelines in psychiatry. We focus on key areas and applications of the clinical intervention and, for scope of this book, are far from exhaustive. To account for the perhaps inevitable diffusion of a clinical intervention, as it flows along the pipeline of implementation, we have deemed it necessary (and justified) to orient at times around both available clinical efficacy and effectiveness literature as well as what we perceive is real-world, common belief and practice. Elsewhere, we offer possible alternative interpretations of established findings in order to remind the reader of the potential for subjectivity when drawing clinical inference from certain study designs. We suggest that it is what we hold true as field at large, not the raw sum of the literature, that principally drives real-world patient outcomes. We nevertheless trust that the reader will critically consider the evidence and assertions in this work through their own lens of experience and expertise.

Writing this book has itself been an exercise in shared decision-making. The process sparked numerous controversies among the three of us, followed by discussions that led us to repeatedly reexamine our own prescribing behaviors and identities as mental health professionals. It facilitated a consideration of the wide socioeconomic context of the practice of psychopharmacology as well as the individual patient's experience. Most importantly, it led each of us down an inward path that was defined by our individual culture, upbringing, belief systems, and medical, psychiatric, and psychological training. Rather than attempting to expunge these differences and present this book as a standard, uniform guideline, we briefly elucidate our individual training and the experiences that affect our understanding and practices around psychopharmacology.

Swapnil Gupta was born and brought up in the small town of Pondicherry, in Southern India. She went to a medical school that highlighted critical engagement with the pharmaceutical industry, close examination of evidence-based treatments, and rational use of medical testing, medications, and other interventions. In her psychiatric residencies in both India and the United States, she encountered patients whose psychological suffering was equally related to economic, sexual, racial, and various forms of disenfranchisement as it was to diagnosable mental disorders. In her clinical practice, she attempts to maintain a complex, biopsychosocial view of her patients' experience, at every stage of their treatment. For her, this book is a combination of rational medication use, critical evaluation of the available evidence base, parsimonious and equitable use of resources, and, finally, making the patient's voice heard.

Rebecca Miller grew up in New Jersey, in the United States, as part of a white, upper middle-class protestant family. Her quest to understand her own experiences with mental illness and the mental health system led her to obtain a degree in clinical psychology and to work in community mental health in order to help create a more equitable mental health system. She directs peer support and trains psychiatry residents and psychology interns, incorporating her lived experience into her efforts to improve mental health care. The effort around deprescribing is, for her, a civil rights endeavor, in support of others interested in trying the "experiment" of reducing or stopping medications in an empowered, collaborative way.

John D. Cahill was raised in the United Kingdom and has a bi-cultural background, having been exposed to both Western and Eastern perspectives on wellness. He felt a calling as a physician from a young age, attended medical school during the ascent of evidence-based medicine, biological psychiatry and community-based mental health care, and moved to the United States for specialty training, drawn by opportunities for innovation of psychiatric care. His work spans biomarker and new drug target development, the psychotherapeutic aspects of prescribing, and building learning healthcare systems. His principle occupation remains the care of individuals with both emerging and persisting serious mental illness. Struck by the inherent (and at times meaningful) uncertainty and imprecision within psychiatric care—and the range of reactions (for better or for worse) one might manifest to this challenge (from patients, caregivers, providers, academia, care systems, government, and society as a whole), he is honored to contribute to this book principally to illuminate the issues, offer a starting point for deprescribing practice and frame questions for future research and debate. John does not presume that deprescribing will result in psychopharmacology becoming less prominent in psychiatry, but that deprescribing represents a meaningful construct for all stakeholders to consider in order to ensure minimum-effective dosing of medications and robust therapeutic alliance.

—SG, RM, JC

New Haven, CT

April, 2019

Acknowledgments

This book acknowledges our patients - past, present and future - who teach us so much. It is also the culmination of influences from so many teachers, mentors, family, and friends, each of whom added their voice in different ways to the thinking represented in this book. We wish we could acknowledge each of them individually as they have contributed so much to the development of this book and provided the support to allow for the time it took in the writing.

The work described in this book was funded in part by the State of Connecticut, Department of Mental Health and Addiction Services (DMHAS), but this publication does not express the views of DMHAS or the State of Connecticut. The views and opinions expressed are those of the authors. We are grateful to DMHAS for the support it provides for this work.

In particular we want to express gratitude to Michael Sernyak, Robert Cole and Jeanne Steiner at the Connecticut Mental Health Center (CMHC) for providing the space and support to work in innovative ways; the people receiving services at CMHC, who inspire us with their strength and courage and honor us by sharing their stories with us; Megan Katz, for her keen editorial eye and broad vision for the organization of the book; Yaara Zisman-Ilani, John Strauss, and Vinod Srihari, for comments on the manuscript; and Sandy Steingard and Tamar Lavy, who have shared countless thoughts, ideas, and stories.

Thank you to our editors at Oxford University Press; Andrea Knobloch and Lani Oshima, as well as assistants Allison Pratt and Ann Sanchez, for their patience and support in this process.

In addition, SG owes a debt of gratitude to her parents (Yogi and Alka), teachers at JIPMER and PGIMER, Stephen Goldfinger, Nina Schooler, Mohini Ranganathan, and Deepak Cyril D'Souza, her wonderful team of clinicians at CMHC (Candace, Dorothy, Laurie, Melissa, Molly, Monica, Terri). RM would like to acknowledge and thank Erika Carr, Allison Ponce, Michelle Silva, and Christy Olezeski for stalwart support and positive peer pressure; the peer support team at CMHC; Larry Davidson, Janis Tondora,

Chyrell Bellamy, Michael Rowe, Anthony Pavlo and others at Program for Recovery and Community Health, for their inspiring work; and family ASM, KSM, DHM. JC would like to specifically acknowledge the mentorship of the late Ralph Hoffman, whose brilliance and humanity was a shining example for the field. JC is indebted to collaborators and mentors at the University of Nottingham, the University of Huddersfield, and Yale University, and for funding support (of separate, but informing work) from the National Institutes of Health, the Brain & Behavior Research Foundation, the Rabinowitz family, and the Patrick and Catherine Weldon Donaghue Medical Research Foundation.

—SG, RM, JC

PART 1
THE CONTEXT
FOR DEPRESCRIBING

1

Deprescribing in Psychiatry

An Introduction

This chapter provides the foundation for the rest of the book, defining the concept of deprescribing and relating it specifically to working with the deprescribing of medications in psychiatry. It provides a rationale and history of the concept of deprescribing, outlines the potential benefits of adapting deprescribing to psychiatry, and orients the reader to the rest of the content of the book.

Goal and Learning Objectives

After reading this chapter, the reader will be able to:

1. Define the concept of deprescribing
2. Give three justifications for its application in psychiatry
3. Identify three ways in which deprescribing is congruent with recovery-oriented care

Deprescribing as a Critical Intervention in Psychiatry

Psychiatry is at a crossroads, one where the overmedicalization of distress, economic interests of 'Big Pharma', and soaring health care costs intersect with the promise of more effective and precise biological treatments. Although the introduction of newer psychotropic medications has expanded the treatment options in psychiatry, there is a risk of overprescription and unrealistic expectations in terms of risk–benefit ratios. For instance, psychotropic medications such as fluoxetine (Prozac), quetiapine (Seroquel), and aripiprazole (Abilify) have made the blockbuster medication list on several occasions in the past two decades. However, they have also been the subject of scrutiny around side effects, resulting in major class action lawsuits against their manufacturers. This warrants careful reexamination of current prescription practices and a recalibration of our understanding of the potential risks and benefits of prescribing psychotropic medications for a given condition or symptom.

Every individual is a stakeholder in the public debate surrounding the issue of psychiatric medications, but this debate is exceptionally significant to individuals experiencing distress, their families, and the people who work in mental health, including psychiatrists, nurse practitioners, pharmacists, psychologists, social workers, allied caregivers and physicians in other specialties.

Alongside this is the emergence of the voices of people with the illness, including radical groups who contend that the experiences termed mental illness are an extension of the range of human experience and not to be pathologized. The social contexts of community breakdown, poverty, racism, and discrimination against a range of identity markers, along with the resultant trauma, can feed a widespread rejection of strict biological explanations for the psychological distress that the individual faces.

Deprescribing is one avenue for addressing this expansion of drug prescription and the medicalization of distress. While certainly not a panacea, we believe that the expanded deprescribing intervention described in this book has the potential to help shift practice by acknowledging the inherent uncertainties in psychiatric treatments and by guiding prescribers in working collaboratively in (de)prescribing psychotropic medications. We use the structure of deprescribing to frame and address the questions of balancing risks with benefits, patient autonomy with community interests, and medical expertise with experiential expertise.

A Definition

Scott et al. (2015) defined "deprescribing" as the "reduction or cessation of potentially inappropriate medications in situations where existing or potential risks outweigh existing or potential benefit, taking into consideration the patient's medical and functional status and preferences". In this way it can be regarded as a *collaborative inquiry, within a shared decision-making framework, toward the goal of minimum effective medication usage.* It is neither an "anti-prescribing" stance, nor a denial or invalidation of suffering, nor a rejection of evidence-based treatment. The term "deprescribing" was originally coined in geriatric medicine, where patients are at greater risk for serious consequences of polypharmacy due to side effects, additive effects and ensuing drug–drug interactions. This risk escalates in patients as they age, in part because of altered metabolism of medications as well as because of the increasing incidence of polypharmacy. In the geriatric population, the potential negative consequences of polypharmacy have included increased falls, altered mental status, and cardiac arrhythmias (Woodward, 2003). The highly visible impact of polypharmacy in geriatric patients may have functioned as the proverbial "canary in the coal mine," making the danger readily apparent and visible to all. This most vulnerable population inspired a movement toward reevaluating medication regimens, one that has pushed the field of geriatric medicine into defining prompts, protocols, and guidelines for implementing deprescribing (e.g., the Beers Criteria; Fick & Semla, 2012).

Since then, deprescribing is increasingly emerging in other medical specialties, including cardiology, in which, recently, the idea of the long-term use of various medications including aspirin, statins, beta-blockers, and angiotensin converting enzyme inhibitors following a myocardial infarction has also been called into question (Rossello, Pocock & Julian, 2015). The lack of clear evidence for guidelines around their continued use, along with concerns regarding polypharmacy and a lack of trials on drug withdrawal have continued to motivate this work. In primary care, proton pump inhibitors have become a target of deprescribing as the data on long-term efficacy are increasingly being recognized as inadequate (Boghossian et al., 2017; Reeve et al., 2015; Walsh et al., 2016). In neurology, research in epilepsy has established the feasibility and advantages of discontinuing anticonvulsant medications, particularly for those who have not had seizures for a given period of time (Aktekin et al., 2006; Dash et al., 2015). Guidelines have now emerged to specify those patients for whom deprescribing antiepileptic drugs is recommended (Beghi et al., 2013). Our work takes this argument forward into the mental health realm, where the serious potential consequences of long-term psychotropic usage (such as increase cardiovascular mortality) need to be weighed against benefits and patient preference (Parks et al., 2006).

The limited frequency of review of risk/benefit ratios in chronic pharmacotherapy is an unfortunate result of real-world practice across all medical specialties. Factors influencing this may include an inadequate evidence base for the required duration of pharmacotherapy and an absence of trials on how to discontinue a medication. Furthermore, adjusting or reducing medications may provoke fear of "rocking the boat" if a patient has attained medical stability with some difficulty (Steinman & Landefeld, 2018). Prescribers may also feel an obligation to do "something" when faced with a person's suffering, biasing them toward continuing to prescribe the same or additional medications. Although well-meaning, this risks violating the basic tenet of "first, do no harm," when the continued use of a medication results in more negative than positive effects.

Medicine has been said to be vulnerable to the "therapeutic illusion," which is a tendency to attribute improvement or recovery to medical interventions even though there may be other factors that may partially or completely explain an improvement (Casarett, 2016; Thomas, 1978). For instance, a physician who prescribes an antidepressant to a depressed patient may attribute any resulting improvement in symptoms to the medication. The reality may be that the patient presented toward the tail-end of the natural course of the episode (an untreated episode of depression is expected to last 6–9 months); that the patient stopped drinking alcohol at the same time as starting medication; or that the patient experienced a significant social context change (such as getting a new job or starting a new relationship).

Although the concept of deprescribing can easily become entangled in deep philosophical, social, political, and ethical debate, at the core of deprescribing (and this work) is a structured, multifaceted clinical intervention warranting further development, study, and dissemination. While relatively well-developed in geriatric medicine, this intervention has only recently emerged in psychiatry. It is crucial to differentiate the intervention of deprescribing from the mere act of 'discontinuation' or 'withdrawal' of psychotropic medications which have been variable defined, implemented and studied in psychiatry.

Why Psychiatry Needs Deprescribing

The concepts of shared decision-making, minimum effective dosing, and medication discontinuation research are not new to psychiatry. However, with the relatively greater emphasis on medication initiation and continuation in clinical literature, guidelines, and training, the option of medication reduction may be easily overlooked. Organizing the approach and

furthering research around the construct of deprescribing may help to re-
dress this imbalance. We elaborate reasons why deprescribing is critical to
psychiatry, focusing on the preservation of patient autonomy, minimization of polypharmacy, and the contextualization of reductionistic biological
models.

Patient Autonomy

The topic of the ethics of psychiatry has been extensively written about
in books, papers and the like. Patient autonomy is particularly pertinent to deprescribing due to its foundation in shared decision making.
Psychiatry's past may continue to reverberate in negative ways and psychiatric providers would do well to acknowledge the past history of the
field, which has included the implementation of later-proven-ineffective or
even harmful treatments prior to the more wide-spread adoption of medical research ethics committees and evidenced-based medicine. Included
in these are such practices as cold-packing, lobotomy, and insulin-induced
coma—the images of which contribute to current stigmatization of both the
field and our patients. Some of the patients currently seen in our mental
health systems have had personal experiences with these therapies. Could
deprescribing be an opportunity to heal the iatrogenic trauma and mis-
trust which lingers from not too distant past? Whilst being a far from
straightforward issue, involuntary commitment, the use of restraints, and
legally mandated medication continue to be regular practices in the face
of emergent or imminent risk, along with more subtle forms of coercion
which erode patient autonomy. Practices that undermine trust and decrease
perceived and actual patient autonomy around treatment decisions become
especially problematic if procedural justice is not served. Deprescribing, as
an intervention in psychiatry, is conceptualized as one that stands to increase patient autonomy.

Deprescribing as a Biopsychosocial Intervention

Although the psychiatry mainstream has prided itself on maintaining a
"biopsychosocial" approach to its disorders and treatment, biomedical
explanations and treatments have overshadowed psychological and social

interventions in recent decades. With its greater emphasis on psychotherapeutic and social supports, deprescribing offers an opportunity and
framework to rebalance the biopsychosocial approach to the treatment of
psychiatric disorders while bringing together key care stakeholders in a collaborative mode. For example, when an antipsychotic medication is reduced
to a minimum effective dose within the framework of deprescribing, this
may lead to an increased investment in social supports, lifestyle changes, and
psychotherapeutic interventions. Ensuring that treatment does not become
"toxic help" is an imperative in providing responsible, ethical, and effective
care in psychiatry (Deegan & Drake, 2006). The availability of deprescribing
could serve as a safeguard to ensure that the use of medications are limited
to situations in which they are clearly indicated; to reorient and rebalance
the focus of treatment to psychological and social factors (see Figure 1.1);
and to promote collaboration with the patient as an equal partner in his or
her own care.

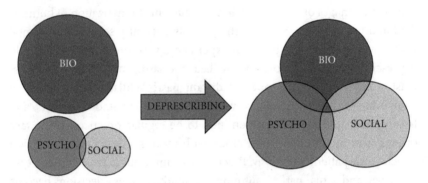

Figure 1.1 Increased integration and balance of bio-psycho-social approaches
as a collateral benefit of deprescribing. The scenario on the left represents a
patient's treatment, where a prescriber is addressing some medical health
factors and prescribing several medications. The prescriber is working in
relative isolation from a therapist who is addressing both psychological and
social factors with the patient (however, overall, and in the eyes of the patient,
the major focus is on the pharmacotherapy). The prescriber and patient initiate
a deprescribing of one medication—involving the therapist from the outset.
This promotes the scenario on the right, where there is increased collaboration
between providers and psychosocial factors become more prominent in the
patient's treatment.

Nonconcordance

Many patients already seek to discontinue their medications and may do so on their own regardless of their prescriber's advice or involvement. The adherence rates to medication in schizophrenia provides one illustration, with reported rates ranging from 42% to 95% (Sendt et al., 2015). Could proactively addressing the option of reducing or stopping medications preempt risks surrounding patient-initiated, abrupt medication discontinuation? When requested by a patient, who with capacity, is aware of the risks, the outstanding question for the prescriber becomes not *whether* to guide a therapeutically optimal discontinuation, but instead determining *how*. The focus on the doctor–patient relationship, building trust, and maintaining communication and connection is an essential element of all medicine but becomes particularly highlighted in deprescribing. In this way deprescribing can promote concordance between prescriber and patient.

Deprescribing as a Recovery-Oriented Practice

Our understanding of recovery-oriented practice does not mandate the universal deprescribing of psychotropic medications. However the rationale for deprescribing in psychiatry fall within the related overarching concept of *recovery-oriented care* that links them philosophically. The idea that someone with a mental illness can live a meaningful life, pursuing important life goals, was seen as a somewhat radical notion in the late twentieth century but has since taken hold as a dominant paradigm in the United States and internationally in recent years. The idea that people can live with and live beyond their psychological symptoms provides a challenge to previous conceptualizations of mental illness as a sort of "life sentence." Deprescribing (like de-institutionalization and de-hospitalization) seems like a natural progression in the evolution of thinking about mental illness—one that takes into consideration the lived experience of those of us (including co-author RM) who live with mental illness or experiences of extreme emotional distress. Baker et al. (2013) argue for the reorganizing of the psychiatrist–patient relationship to better orient medication prescribing with recovery-based principles. In line with person-centered principles, the patient is encouraged and educated about being a full partner in decisions around medication and other treatments (see Figure 1.2).

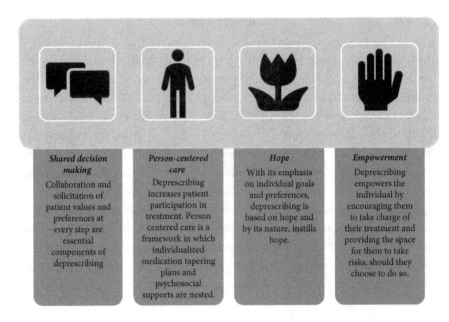

Shared decision making	Person-centered care	Hope	Empowerment
Collaboration and solicitation of patient values and preferences at every step are essential components of deprescribing	Deprescribing increases patient participation in treatment. Person centered care is a framework in which individualized medication tapering plans and psychosocial supports are nested.	With its emphasis on individual goals and preferences, deprescribing is based on hope and by its nature, instills hope.	Deprescribing empowers the individual by encouraging them to take charge of their treatment and providing the space for them to take risks, should they choose to do so.

Figure 1.2 Deprescribing is well-aligned with recovery-oriented principles.

Shared decision-making has been identified as one of the key practices in deprescribing (cf. Miller & Pavlo, 2018). Principles such as respect for patient autonomy and viewing the person as an expert in his or her own experience, including that of illness and health, support the conceptualization of deprescribing as a recovery-oriented practice. In addition, the focus of treatment shifts from clinical recovery to personal recovery, which means that, instead of having a specific symptom-related goal, treatment is modified to suit the patient's attitudes, values, and life goals. Deprescribing, with its focus on the patient's values, attitudes, and preferences, is an intervention that espouses personal recovery. Table 1.1 identifies specific recovery-oriented practices and how they apply to deprescribing.

A key element of recovery-oriented care is the use of person-first language and descriptions that are empowering. Referring to someone as "noncompliant" or "lacking insight" (1) is not behaviorally anchored, (2) suggests judgment of behavior (as opposed to value-free observation), and (3) implies a lack of autonomy on behalf of the patient. We encourage paying special attention to the language used while discussing and documenting deprescribing. In the spirit of recognizing patients' expertise

Table 1.1 Some recovery-oriented practices in mental health and their application to deprescribing

Practice	Description	Application to deprescribing
Shared decision-making (Davidson, Tondora, Pavlo, & Stanhope, 2017; Deegan & Drake, 2006)	SDM is a process of collaboration to arrive at a mutually acceptable plan for moving forward in the treatment process. It involves two experts: the physician with scientific and clinical knowledge, and the person who knows his or her own preferences, values, and subjective experiences.	Collaboration, provision of education, and solicitation of the patient's preferences and values at every step are essential components of deprescribing
Person-centered care (Davidson et al., 2017; Stanhope, Ingoglia, Schmelter, & Marcus, 2013; Tondora, Miller, Slade, & Davidson, 2014)	Person-centered care puts the person receiving care in the driver's seat, and focuses on life goals vs. treatment goals. It is a highly individual comprehensive approach to developing a care plan for achieving life goals rather than a problem focus or strictly symptom relief.	Deprescribing aims to increase quality of life via reducing use of medications as applicable. Person-centered care offers a framework in which individualized tapering plans as well as psychosocial supports are nested.
Hope (Jacobson & Greenley, 2001)	Hope is the belief that recovery is possible. High expectations and a belief that a person can achieve goals is crucial to recovery.	With its emphasis on individual goals and preferences, deprescribing potentially instills hope.
Empowerment (Jacobson & Greenley, 2001)	Empowerment may be viewed as a corrective for learned helplessness and low self-efficacy that may have been instilled by the mental health system. It includes autonomy, courage and responsibility.	Engaging in the process of deprescribing may empower the individual by encouraging them to take charge of their treatment and providing the space for them to take risks, should they choose to do so.

and their right and ability to make decisions (whether we agree or not) for themselves, it is essential to use respectful, recovery-oriented language.

Deprescribing Provides a Systematic Way to Address Irrational Polypharmacy

Polypharmacy (both rational and irrational) has increased in a substantial way over the past decade. When defined as the use of five or more prescription drugs, polypharmacy across all drugs increased from an estimated 8.2% in 1999–2000 to 15% in 2011–2012 in the United States (Kantor et al., 2015).

Although some data support the use of combinations of individual antidepressants and antipsychotic medications, the duration for which combinations should be used is unknown (Dodd et al., 2005; Freudenreich & Goff, 2002). In their review, Stahl and Grady (2004) observed that most investigators did not try to discontinue one of the drugs after the combination proved beneficial to establish a true need for the combination. This practice of continuing medications unchanged without a clear understanding of their necessity can lead to drug interactions and serious side effects, often without any benefit. Deprescribing prompts prescribers and patients to periodically reassess the risks and benefits of each medication and provides a framework within which to implement reduction and/or cessation of medications considered redundant or for which the risks may outweigh the benefits.

Prescribing and Deprescribing as a Complex Intervention

Prescribing and deprescribing medications, despite mechanistic models would have us believe, are not simple endeavors; they qualify as complex interventions for complex problems, particularly in psychiatry. Glouberman and Zimmerman (2002) compare and contrast approaches to simple, complicated, and complex problems in health care, using the respective metaphors of cooking a recipe, launching a rocket, and raising a child (see Table 1.2). A *simple* problem can be addressed with a basic set of procedures with predictable results; a *complicated* problem requires more expertise, but results nevertheless have high degree of certainty.

Table 1.2 Comparing the approach to simple, complicated, and complex problems

Approaching Simple, Complicated, vs. Complex Problems		
Simple: *Following a recipe*	**Complicated:** *Sending a rocket to the moon*	**Complex:** *Raising a child*
The recipe is essential	Formulas are critical and necessary	Formulas have a limited application
Recipes are tested to assure easy replication	Sending one rocket increases assurance that the next will be OK	Raising one child provides experience but no assurance of success with the next
No particular expertise is required. But cooking expertise increases success rate	High levels of expertise in a variety of fields are necessary for success	Expertise can contribute but is neither necessary nor sufficient to assure success
Recipes produce standardized products	Rockets are similar in critical ways	Every child is unique and must be understood as an individual
The best recipes give good results every time	There is a high degree of certainty of outcome	Uncertainty of outcome remains
Optimistic approach to problem possible	Optimistic approach to problem possible	Optimistic approach to problem possible

From Glouberman & Zimmerman (2002) and University of Toronto Press (2004). Reprinted with permission of the publisher.

When addressing *complex* problems, however, formulas, procedures, and expertise do not guarantee success and uncertainty abounds. This distinction can be usefully applied to prescribing and deprescribing in psychiatry.

Despite what our neurobiological models would have us believe, the act of prescribing a medication is best regarded as a complex intervention. Effecting antagonism at dopaminergic D_2 receptors in the mesolimbic pathway with haloperidol, on a receptor level, could indeed be regarded as a simple problem. However, when the problem is framed on the level of attempting to care for an individual's experiencing a psychotic disorder with said medication, the picture becomes more complex. Individual differences in pharmacokinetics and dynamics, nonlinear dose–response effects, heterogeneity, and uncertainties in the pathoetiology of the psychotic experiences, the level of the patient's concordance, sense of meaning and understanding of the recommended prescription and access (e.g., insurance coverage) to the medication potentially interact to confound the desired result. The interacting factors grow exponentially when adding in the psychosocial context, culture, history of the individual, and relationship between prescriber and patient—to identify a few, but certainly not all, confounding variables.

For better or worse, trials of drug efficacy attempt to render this complexity more manageable with stringent research methods (e.g. study protocols, the checking of drug levels, and objective markers of target engagement). However, when generalized into real-world effectiveness, the waters are inevitably muddied, and implementation science readily recognizes the resultant gap in knowledge translation. Accordingly, while engaging a patient in shared decision-making around pharmacotherapy, it is vital to also engage in an individualized, flexible, responsive, multiperspective approach, one that optimistically acknowledges uncertainty and ever-changing bio-psycho-social-cultural factors.

To use the aforementioned metaphor, a parent persisting with the same child-rearing strategies successful at 2-year-old when the child is 15 may be disappointed. To assume (without confirmatory evidence) a static system (i.e. a given pharmacotherapy will continue to work indefinitely for an individual) may be over-simplifying. In this way, psychiatry must be armed with research and guidelines for both starting and stopping medications until we have clear justification to the contrary.

Settings for Deprescribing

In today's health care systems, primary care physicians are especially well-positioned to implement deprescribing as they coordinate with different specialties for a given patient. Typical settings in which psychiatric medications are prescribed include primary care, geriatric clinics, nursing homes, public sector or community mental health centers, private practices, intensive outpatient programs, and inpatient services (acute and long-term). These may include state-funded agencies, nonprofits, Veterans Affairs (VA) hospitals, private clinics, and combinations of these. Ideally, deprescribing would require infrastructure that would facilitate reliable communication between providers from different specialties. This would include electronic medical records (EMR) with updated medication lists accessible by multiple providers and secure messaging facilities. Accessibility to other supports, such as groups and individual therapy and drug and alcohol treatments, may be necessary in certain cases. For instance, the VA hospital system has patients seeing multiple medical specialists at the same location with a single medical record containing a consolidated list of medications. In this situation, the primary care physician is well-placed to initiate a conversation about deprescribing, both with the providers from various specialties and with the patient; although the deprescribing should ultimately be conducted by the prescriber who initiated and manages the target medication.

In public-sector agencies, the coordination of treatments for mental and physical disorders has been a challenge when such services are obtained at different locations and sometimes even when they are co-located at the same facility. To address this issue, the Substance Abuse and Mental Health Services Administration and the Health Resources and Services Administration (SAMHSA-HRSA) Center for Integrated Health Solutions has developed one version of what has become known as a *behavioral health home,* with the goal of coordinating all health services that a given individual needs either in-house or using a co-located partnership model (Alexander & Druss, 2012). Two of the core principles of effective care at these health homes are patient-centered care and evidence-based care. As the goal of these health homes is coordination and patient-centered care, with decision support as a core principle, they may form an ideal location for the implementation of a deprescribing initiative. On inpatient psychiatric units, patients who have not responded to various combinations of medications may be deprescribed all their medications to make a "fresh start"—something not always feasible on an outpatient basis, especially for those with a history of severe illness and high potential for imminent risk. In this setting, deprescribing may be carried out more rapidly because the purpose is not merely the reduction of side effects but the identification of a helpful medication.

Deprescribing may also be offered as a "consultation service" to the primary treating team. A consultation team that is able to conduct detailed history and medication review, assess the likelihood of relapse, measure and treat withdrawal symptoms, and suggest alternatives to medication as part of a detailed deprescribing plan may be a more feasible way of implementing deprescribing in large systems. The team would ideally include a pharmacist and an internist who could weigh in on side effects and interactions.

This process may be conducted as a quality-improvement or utilization review initiative.

The Ethics of Deprescribing

It is unfeasible in this intended pragmatic book to adequately review the ethics of deprescribing. Autonomy and non-maliference have already been mentioned. Nevertheless, it is easy to imagine the relevance of all ethical prinicples to a given deprescribing decision. Repeated reviews of medication lists ensure that medications do not end up causing more harm than good (nonmaleficence) and that the treatment that is offered is truly beneficial (beneficence). In mental illness, the struggle between individual (autonomy) and societal (justice) interests risks being resolved at the expense of the individual's autonomy. Mandated and coercive treatments are justified by citing poor insight and/or judgment in combination with perceived risk to or even burden on society. There is a risk that deprescribing may be viewed as an error of omission or as a withholding of appropriate services. To offset this risk, it is crucial to remain aware of potential ethical dilemas related to deprescribing, both as prescribers and as a field.

Conclusion

This chapter presents the initial description of how to conceptualize and begin thinking about the issues related to the implementation and study of deprescribing in psychiatry. We see this intervention as *more than just medication adjustment*; it is a holistic expansion in approach and techniques relevant to both the reduction *and initiation* of medications, one geared toward promoting recovery for individuals diagnosed with mental illness.

While in other medical conditions the reduction or elimination of medication use may be more straightforward, we contend that mental illness is not "an illness like any other," does not yet neatly map onto a clear pathophysiology like diabetes or hypertension, and does not equate simply to something like the reduction of a statin for hypercholesterolemia. For historical, cultural, and inter- and intra-personal reasons, psychiatric medications have a much greater meaning, impact, symbolism, and potential risk related to their reduction or discontinuation. Mental illness affects one's core sense of being, one's interpersonal relationships, and one's potential ability to move forward in life. Along with a history of psychiatry that has more recently heavily emphasized the medical model over social or alternative explanations of illness, each of these sociocultural factors highlights the need for a more complex and multifaceted approach to pharmacotherapy. Drawing from and complementing the recovery literature in mental health, deprescribing in psychiatry is a potential venue for achieving the ultimate goal of psychiatry: decreasing human suffering.

Our audience for this book includes interested professionals who prescribe psychiatric medications, including primary care physicians, psychiatrists, advanced practical nurses, psychologists, physician associates and others. Interested allied professionals including pharmacists, social workers, peer support, administrators, and policymakers may find the ideas useful in helping to reorganize existing services to be more recovery-oriented. We also imagine that patients and their friends and family may be interested in using the book to think through their own process of taking medications, although the intended audience is primarily professionals and more specifically prescribers.

On this note, we wish to address the use of the term "prescriber" in this book. Despite some controversy over the use of the term, we chose "prescriber" to refer to the person prescribing the medication, including psychiatrists, nurse practitioners, psychologists, physicians' associates, trainees, and physicians in other specialties. We decided to use this term to describe the person writing the prescription for both expediency and inclusivity. We clearly advocate that the value of a "prescriber" not be reduced to the act of writing a prescription.

This book is geared to support learning about the considerations to address when introducing deprescribing. The next chapter discusses the complex process of decision-making in psychiatry and how that relates to deprescribing process. Chapter 3 identifies and describes barriers to deprescribing and what can be done to overcome them. Chapter 4 addresses some of the psychological considerations when deprescribing, identifying the meaning of the medication and other factors that demand to be addressed. Chapter 5 outlines the various supports and strategies that a patient can access on his or her own in order to support deprescribing. Chapter 6 continues in this vein, discussing interventions that a prescriber or clinician may recommend adding to a range of services in order to best support deprescribing. Chapter 7 outlines each step of deprescribing and elaborates on considerations for decision-making. Chapters 8–11 address specific classes of psychotropic medication (antidepressant, antipsychotic, mood stabilizers, benzodiazepines, and stimulants) and the considerations around deprescribing these. Chapter 12 is a summary and offers future directions for this emerging and important area of psychiatric practice.

Each chapter contains specific learning objectives, case examples, and a self-assessment to monitor reader understanding. We hope this book provides guidance and thought-provoking ideas around the concept of deprescribing as it relates to the broader trajectory of transforming mental health care to be recovery-oriented and person-centered.

Self-Assessment

1. **Deprescribing as an intervention can encompass**
   a. Medication reduction and/or discontinuation
   b. Consultation with primary care physicians, pharmacists, and specialists
   c. Consultation with the patient and his or her support system
   d. The medication regimen ultimately remaining the same
   e. All of the above

   Correct answer: e.

2. **Which of the following is not an indication for initiating deprescribing in psychiatry?**
   a. Patient preference
   b. Side effects and drug interactions
   c. No clear demonstration of therapeutic benefit
   d. Request from the patient's significant other

   Correct answer: d.

3. **Which of the following is a recovery-based practice espoused by deprescribing?**
   a. Beneficence
   b. Empowerment
   c. Autonomy
   d. Nonmaleficence

   Correct answer: b.

References

Aktekin, B., Dogan, E. A., Oguz, Y., & Senol, Y. (2006). Withdrawal of antiepileptic drugs in adult patients free of seizures for 4 years: A prospective study. *Epilepsy & Behavior, 8*(3), 616–619.

Alexander, L., & Druss, B. (2012). *Behavioral Health Homes for People with Mental Health and Substance Use Conditions: The Core Clinical Features.* Washington, DC: SAMHSA-HRSA Center for Integrated Health Solutions, US Department of Health and Human Services.

Baker, E., Fee, J., Bovingdon, L., Campbell, T., Hewis, E., Lewis, D., . . . Roberts, G. (2013). From taking to using medication: recovery-focused prescribing and medicines management. *Advances in Psychiatric Treatment, 19*(1), 2–10.

Beghi, E., Giussani, G., Grosso, S., Iudice, A., Neve, A. L., Pisani, F., . . . Michelucci, R. (2013). Withdrawal of antiepileptic drugs: guidelines of the Italian League Against Epilepsy. *Epilepsia, 54*(s7), 2–12.

Boghossian, T. A., Rashid, F. J., Thompson, W., Welch, V., Moayyedi, P., Rojas-Fernandez, C., . . . Farrell, B. (2017). Deprescribing versus continuation of chronic proton pump inhibitor use in adults. *The Cochrane Library.*

Casarett, D. (2016). The science of choosing wisely: Overcoming the therapeutic illusion. *New England Journal of Medicine, 374*(13), 1203–1205. doi: 10.1056/NEJMp1516803.

Davidson, L., Tondora, J., Pavlo, A. J., & Stanhope, V. (2017). Shared decision making within the context of recovery-oriented care. *Mental Health Review Journal, 22*(3), 179–190.

Deegan, P. E., & Drake, R. E. (2006). Shared decision making and medication management in the recovery process. *Psychiatric Services, 57*(11), 1636–1639.

Dodd, S., Horgan, D., Malhi, G. S., & Berk, M. (2005). To combine or not to combine? A literature review of antidepressant combination therapy. *Journal of Affective Disorders, 89*(1–3), 1–11.

Drake, R. E., & Deegan, P. E. (2009). Shared decision making is an ethical imperative. *Psychiatric Services, 60*(8), 1007.

Fick, D. M., & Semla, T. P. (2012). 2012 American Geriatrics Society Beers Criteria: New year, new criteria, new perspective. *Journal of the American Geriatrics Society, 60*(4), 614–615.

Freudenreich, O., & Goff, D. (2002). Antipsychotic combination therapy in schizophrenia. A review of efficacy and risks of current combinations. *Acta Psychiatrica Scandinavica, 106*(5), 323–330.

Glouberman, S., & Zimmerman, B. (2002). Complicated and complex systems: What would successful reform of Medicare look like? *Romanow Papers*, *2*, 21–53.

Gupta, S., & Cahill, J. D. A prescription for "deprescribing" in psychiatry. *Psychiatric Services*, *67*(8). doi: 10.1176/appi.ps.201500359.

Gupta, S., Cahill, J. D., & Miller, R. (2018). Deprescribing antipsychotics: A guide for clinicians. *British Journal of Psychiatric Advances*, *24*(5), 295–302.

Jacobson, N., & Greenley, D. (2001). What is recovery? A conceptual model and explication. *Psychiatric Services*, *52*(4), 482–485.

Kantor, E. D., Rehm, C. D., Haas, J. S., Chan, A. T., & Giovannucci, E. L. (2015). Trends in prescription drug use among adults in the united states from 1999–2012. *JAMA*, *314*(17), 1818–1830. doi: 10.1001/jama.2015.13766.

Miller, R., & Pavlo, A. J. (2018). Two experts, one goal: Collaborative deprescribing in psychiatry. *Current Psychiatry Reviews*, *14*(1), 12–18.

Parks, J., Svendsen, D., Singer, P., Foti, M. E., & Mauer, B. (2006). *Morbidity and Mortality in People with Serious Mental Illness*. Alexandria, VA: National Association of State Mental Health Program Directors (NASMHPD) Medical Directors Council.

Reeve, E., Andrews, J. M., Wiese, M. D., Hendrix, I., Roberts, M. S., & Shakib, S. (2015). Feasibility of a patient-centered deprescribing process to reduce inappropriate use of proton pump inhibitors. *Annals of Pharmacotherapy*, *49*(1), 29–38.

Rossello, X., Pocock, S. J., & Julian, D. G. (2015). Long-term use of cardiovascular drugs: Challenges for research and for patient care. *Journal of the American College of Cardiology*, *66*(11), 1273–1285.

Scott, I. A., Hilmer, S. N., Reeve, E., Potter, K., Le Couteur, D., Rigby, D., ... Page, A. (2015). Reducing inappropriate polypharmacy: The process of deprescribing. *JAMA Internal Medicine*, *175*(5), 827–834.

Sendt, K.-V., Tracy, D. K., & Bhattacharyya, S. (2015). A systematic review of factors influencing adherence to antipsychotic medication in schizophrenia-spectrum disorders. *Psychiatry Research*, *225*(1), 14–30.

Stanhope, V., Ingoglia, C., Schmelter, B., & Marcus, S. C. (2013). Impact of person-centered planning and collaborative documentation on treatment adherence. *Psychiatric Services*, *64*(1), 76–79.

Steinman, M. A., & Landefeld, C. S. (2018). Overcoming inertia to improve medication use and deprescribing. *JAMA*, *320*(18), 1867–1869.

Thomas, K. (1978). The consultation and the therapeutic illusion. *British Medical Journal*, *1*(6123), 1327–1328.

Tondora, J., Miller, R., Slade, M., & Davidson, L. (2014). *Partnering for Recovery in Mental Health: A Practical Guide to Person-Centered Planning*. New York: John Wiley & Sons.

Walsh, K., Kwan, D., Marr, P., Papoushek, C., & Lyon, W. K. (2016). Deprescribing in a family health team: A study of chronic proton pump inhibitor use. *Journal of Primary Health Care, 8*(2), 164–171.

Woodward, M. C. (2003). Deprescribing: Achieving better health outcomes for older people through reducing medications. *Journal of Pharmacy Practice and Research, 33*(4), 323–328.

2

Decision-Making in Deprescribing

The process of making prescribing decisions in psychiatry can be challenging. From equivocal diagnoses and prognoses, to a shifting array of treatment options (with limited precision), all contextualized by a plethora of differing values, preferences, and standards. Both prescriber and patient must face, and operate under, much uncertainty. These decisions are especially difficult when prescriber and patient disagree, when values or preferences conflict with standard guidelines, or simply when no guidelines are available. Looking more closely at *how* to make decisions, and what might support this process, is the focus of this chapter, specifically as it relates to prescribing or deprescribing.

Goal and Learning Objectives

After reading this chapter, the reader will be able to:

1. Better understand a framework for psychopharmacological decision-making
2. Explain a model for the decision-making process in the context of prescribing and deprescribing
3. Gain and apply a greater understanding of one's own decision-making process to provide care that is more sensitive to both scientific evidence and patient preferences
4. Identify the steps of shared decision-making (SDM) and how to create an environment conducive to such

Decision-Making and Decision Analysis

Decision-making is a well-developed science in business management and in medicine. By integrating elements of decision analysis and SDM, this chapter provides us with frameworks to understand why we prescribe what we prescribe, how we reached that decision, and how we can apply this to deprescribing.

Understanding some basic concepts and frameworks in decision-making will enable us to examine our own use of decision-making and to contrast a traditional paternalistic approach with the SDM approach. Traditional decision-making trees end up having limited use in psychiatry due to the relative lack of prediction tools. Even in other branches of medicine where predictive tools, and therefore recommendations, are clearer, there is still growing interest in SDM and greater collaboration towards better person-centered outcomes. We start by reviewing more traditional approaches followed by an expansion on SDM as it specifically applies in psychiatry and deprescribing.

Traditional Decision-Making

A decision is defined as *a conclusion or resolution reached after consideration.* Janis and Mann (1977) defined decision-making as a "cognitive process resulting in the selection of a belief or course of action among several different possibilities" or "the process of identifying and choosing alternatives based on the values and preferences of the decision-maker". Decision analysis is an explicit, quantitative approach to examining difficult decisions about a course of action. It involves the steps of defining the problem, structuring the problem in the form of a decision tree, estimating the uncertainties, and, finally, estimating the relative value of different outcomes - as illustrated in Figure 2.1.

Decision analysis has been applied in medicine to structure and estimate the probability of possible outcomes to a given decision point. In the traditional medical setting, the prescriber–patient interaction entails the patient coming to the prescriber with a complaint that they expect the provider to evaluate, understand, and treat. In general, the prescriber is expected to generate diagnostic possibilities, conduct an interview and examination, and order tests that help narrow down the possibilities and then recommend a treatment that is most likely to address the diagnosis. The process demands the ability to understand (prior) probabilities and make best estimates at several steps, including as it relates to the focus and extent of

SCHEMATIC OF A DECISION TREE

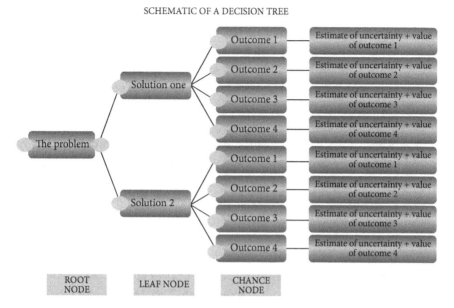

Figure 2.1 Example decision analysis tree schematic.

the history, examination, blood work, and other tests, and hence impacts the recommended treatment. In this way, multiple, parallel decisions are being made implicitly throughout the provider–patient interaction, limiting this kind of single decision analysis.

The preceding clinical process has roots in a traditional paternalistic stance in which the provider is seen as the expert who assesses, analyzes, and decides on the course of treatment, including medications, independent of the patient's values and preferences—to a large degree, *unilateral decision-making*. The provider has the obligation of keeping a patient's best interest in mind as an ethical imperative, but not necessarily including the patient explicitly in the process. While patient preferences may be considered to some extent, there may be little active collaboration, and the provider may still make the decision independently. A medical paternalism model has increasingly lost favor as patients demand more choice and medical information is more widely available and consumed; furthermore, there is a growing body of evidence showing that collaboration between providers and patient can actually improve certain outcomes (Adams & Drake, 2006; Hamann et al., 2003; Wilson et al., 2010).

Facets of Decision-Making

The process of medical decision-making therefore has many facets. The process for both provider and patient often begins before they meet. A prescriber may be influenced by years of training and experience, social and cultural influences, demographic factors, and both conscious and unconscious individual biases. Patients, on the other hand, may have past experiences with certain medications, advice from friends and family, and information about medications through various sources, including advertisements and, increasingly, the internet. The issue of patient complexity, including co-occurring conditions and other variables, has been outlined in a recent model attempting to define this complexity. Through comparing the demands on the patient (e.g., illness burden, socioeconomic factors) with capacity for managing these demands, this newer conceptualization may provide a way of conceiving of patient complexity, but it has not yet been broadly adopted (Shippee, Shah, May, Mair, & Montori, 2012). When patient and provider come together, there is a sharing of information, reasoning, values, and preferences. This sharing is an ongoing process, and prescriber and patient gradually develop a collaborative relationship in the setting of which medication prescriptions can be more finely tuned. It is important to remember that both prescriber and patient have their individual cognitive processes that influence each other and are influenced and refined by the outcome of previous decisions, as illustrated in Figure 2.2.

Applications to Psychiatry

Although extensively used in other fields of interventional medicine, the applicability of decision analysis to psychiatric medication management is limited because of many reasons (summarized in Figure 2.3). Decision analysis and decision-making in psychiatry is challenged by the absence of etiology-based diagnostic systems, lack of diagnostic tests, and imprecision of available treatments. It involves a number of stakeholders, including the prescriber and the patient, but also often family members, spouses, and, in some instances, society in general. In addition to providing relief to the patient, the provider is charged with minimizing risk, both to the patient and to the community. Minimization of risk to the community may come at the expense of violating individual rights, thus generating tension within the

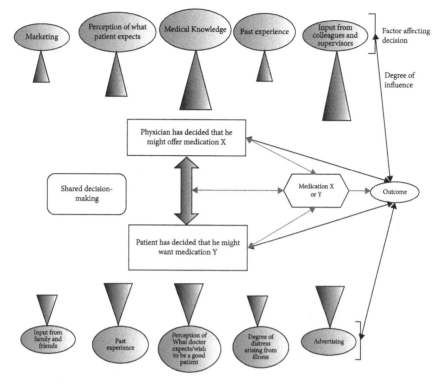

Figure 2.2 Influences on decision-making in the prescriber–patient relationship.

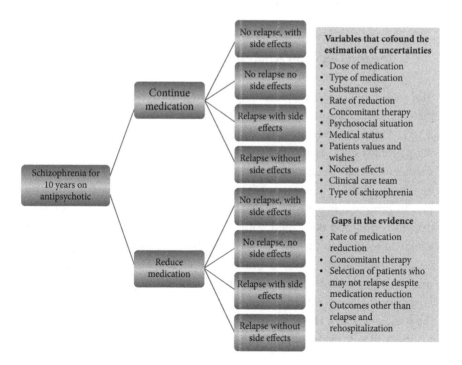

Figure 2.3 Decision analysis in psychiatry.

prescriber themselves and affecting the alliance between the prescriber and the patient.

Psychiatric diagnoses and treatments are uniquely sensitive to sociocultural settings and often bear the burden of a long history of stigma, discrimination, and the history of co-option of psychiatry for social control: for example, the inclusion of homosexuality in the *Diagnostic and Statistical Manual of Mental Disorders* (DSM) or the misuse of psychiatric hospitalization in the oppression of women or political dissidents (Faraone, 1982). Thus, both the macro- and micro-contexts of psychiatric decision-making are composed of constantly changing layers.

Additionally, attaching values to certain outcomes may be complicated. A given patient may highly value being medication-free but may also value staying out of the hospital. Finally, both clinical problems and interventions in psychiatry can be individual, and the evidence base may not have clear answers. Despite these limitations, decision analysis may prove valuable in structuring the problem and systematically examining options, including the evidence base, outcomes, and values, with the overarching goal of minimizing bias toward one course of action (Tavakoli, Davies, & Thomson, 2000). In general though, the movement in medicine more broadly is toward an SDM approach, as outlined in the next section.

Beyond Decision Analysis: Shared Decision-Making

More and more in medicine and in psychiatry, the trend is toward orienting patients and prescribers around collaborative, SDM (Edwards & Elwyn, 2009). Providers are increasingly realizing that the transformation of the patient from a passive recipient of treatment to an active planner and partner in treatment is more likely to lead to outcomes that are desirable to the prescriber–patient team. Shared decision-making is considered a person-centered intervention that respects patient autonomy and self-determination and is a trend going back decades in medicine, while the actual implementation has been slower than hoped (Coylewright et al., 2012; Strull et al., 1984). In the salient scenarios where serious mental illness drives imminent risk, the power to make decisions regarding psychiatric treatments has remained with the prescriber or, in certain cases, with the judicial system. However, this should not impede the default decision-making process moving from "unilateral" to newer models of SDM.

Stages of Decision-Making

The basic framework of SDM identifies three stages during deliberation before a decision: *choice, option,* and *decision* talk. The first stage, *choice talk,* identifies that there is a choice to be made, and the provider conveys this to the patient. This may be clear to the patient prior to meeting (e.g., a patient comes in looking to reduce medications). The second stage, *option talk,* provides further details of treatment options tailored to the patient. The final stage, *decision talk,* encourages an exploration of what matters most to the patient in order to facilitate a decision (Elwyn et al., 2012; Figure 2.4).

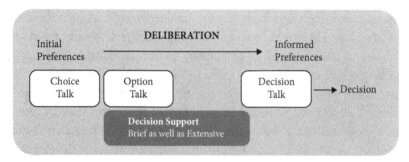

Key to the figure

Deliberation	A process where patients become aware of choice, understand their options and have the time and support to consider 'what matters most to them': may require more than one clinical contact not necessarily face-to-face and may include the use of decision support and discussions with others.
Choice talk	Conveys awareness that a choice exists – initiated by either a patient or a clinician. This may occur before the clinical encounter.
Option talk	Patients are informed about treatment options in more detail.
Decision talk	Patients are supported to explore 'what matters most to them', having become informed.
Decision Support	Decision support as designed in two formats: 1) brief enough to be used by clinician and patient together and 2) more extensive, designed to be used by patients either before or after clinical encounters (paper, DVD, web).
Initial Preferences	Awareness of options leads to the development of initial preferences, based on existing knowledge. The goal is to arrive at informed preferences.
Informed Preferences	Personal preferences based on 'what matters most to patients', predicated on an understanding of the most relevant benefits and harms.

Figure 2.4 Framework of decision-making.
From Elwyn et al. (2012).

Defining the Problem or Identifying a Goal?

In decision analysis, the first step involves identifying a problem and then listing possible treatment options and outcomes. Typically, the problem is formulated in terms of a diagnosis from which the treatment options and outcomes follow. For example, the problem may be hypertension, and the possible treatment options are medication, lifestyle changes, no treatment, or combinations thereof.

An attempt at defining the problem for decision analysis quickly takes us to the heart of the challenge in its application to psychiatry. Is the problem, for instance, treating schizophrenia (or hallucinations) or supporting the person in pursuing a job which they cannot seem to hold on to? What are the barriers to life goals being addressed by the treatment? Ideally, treatments in medicine are expected to be etiology-based: for example, treating tuberculosis with rifampicin, an antibiotic that kills the mycobacteria that cause tuberculosis opposed to a cough suppressant that merely addresses a symptom. Psychiatry is challenged by a lack of treatments that definitively and directly address a defined pathoetiology. Hence, rather than impose presumed treatment/illness-based goals associated with a patient's psychiatric diagnosis, it is prudent to look to the patient to set treatment goals and then present possible treatment options. Literature and the shared expertise of provider and patient can then to some extent inform the possible outcomes.

Drawing from person-centered approaches to care, we can reconceptualize interventions as moving from solely focused on "addressing the problem" to a more positive approach of supporting life goal attainment. Traditionally, care planning starts with the development of a problem list. In person-centered approaches to care, instead, the broader life goal is the focus, with an identification of the barriers standing in the way of goal attainment (Adams & Grieder, 2004; Tondora, Miller, Slade, & Davidson, 2014). These barriers may equally be symptoms treatable by, or side effects caused by, medications. Listening to the functional specifics of each of these barriers is essential in getting a sense of what could be the targets of potential intervention and support.

The first step is hence supporting the person in identifying what they want to change, improve in their life, or move toward. This can be a challenging task for some, as in this chapter's case example of Cindy with her ambivalence about her ability to pursue a job. Other patients may be accustomed to defining their future plans around the circumscribed, institutionalized goals of patienthood, "going to group" and "taking my medications." These are easily spotted as goals imported from previous treaters or, at the very least, the patient's interpretation or internalization of the treaters' expectations. Thus utilizing different and more evocative questions and supporting an exploration either done with the prescriber or allied professional (such as a social worker, peer support specialist, etc.) can better support a fuller understanding of the potential goal and, from that goal, what the choice points may be in terms of treatment.

The SDM stage of *choice talk* helps the patient realize that there are choices available to potentially address identified barriers to achieving their life goals—something that cannot be taken for granted. For example, a patient may be unaware that the fatigue interfering with his job performance could be alleviated by lowering a dose of medication or changing the medication to one that might treat the symptom equally well without causing fatigue. Often, in practice, patients may misattribute a disturbing side effect to one medication and may ask to switch that medication, when the problem may lie with another medication or be an impact of the medication combination. Identifying the choice point and clarifying it to the patient is the first step in deliberations in shared decision-making.

Identifying Alternatives

Once a mutual understanding is reached about what is being addressed and what the hoped outcome will be, the next step is the discussion of possible treatments—*options talk*. As long as a patient is not at imminent danger to themselves or others, and/or is not under legal mandate, the option of not taking any medications is the person's right and needs to be considered as a possible choice even if it may not seem to be the best decision from the prescriber's or others' perspective. For a given symptom configuration, there might be a range of medications available, each in various formulations and doses. When we add medication combinations to the equation, the permutations increase exponentially. Hence, adjustment of doses, formulations, and combinations may be framed as a secondary tool for "fine-tuning" after the initial choice of medication and starting dose is made. In some scenarios this can be overwhelming to both patient and prescriber, who are then at risk of colluding around over-simplified, singular, binary choices. For example, if a patient is doing generally well, the option of increasing dose may be weighed purely against remaining at the same dose, and the option of reducing dose is not generally considered. For patients who have been on the same medication regimen for years, the process of shared decision-making may not have advanced to the stage of identifying all alternatives.

Using decisional support tools such as the Decisional Balance Worksheet (Collins, Carey, & Otto, 2009), the Payoff Matrix from Integrated Treatment for Dual Disorders (Brunette, Drake, & Lynde, 2002), or others can help. These can be completed by either the prescriber and the patient in collaboration, or by the patient prior to an appointment with other clinical staff, peer support staff member, or a family member. Relying on the team approach can increase efficiency and decrease anxiety for the patient as time may be limited in the encounter with the prescriber. Such decisional tools assist people in clearly outlining the cost–benefit ratio or the pros and cons of each decisional option, taking into account a person's values, goals, and preferences.

Choosing Between Alternatives

When the patient–prescriber team generates a set of alternatives, the next step is to zero in on a single, most-valued alternative. This may involve a review of benefits and side effects and viewing those benefits and side effects in the individual patient's context. While choosing between alternatives, the prescriber may use a number of concepts to evaluate and present the information to the patient. The most common framework used to decide on a course of action is the Benefit–Risk Assessment (BRA). BRA is a common decision-making tool employed in medicine. The potential risks of an intervention are weighed against the potential benefits to yield a rough estimate of the risk–benefit ratio. In pharmacoepidemiology, there are several quantitative and qualitative approaches to assessing the BRA but clinically, only a few can be used: Mt-Isa et al. (2014) classify the methodologies as those based on frameworks (such as decision analysis), metric indices (such as quality of life, number needed to treat, tradeoff indices), estimation techniques, and utility survey techniques. It is also important to remember that the relationship between the concepts of risk and benefits is inherently contextual.

In psychiatry, the first difficulty in estimating the risk–benefit ratio is the absence of sufficient information. An attempt at a risk–benefit analysis for a given medication for a given patient at a given point in their life serves to highlight several facts: risk may be dependent on time (a factor that might place a person at risk for an adverse outcome at timepoint A might not do so at timepoint B in the same person); the effect of a risk factor may depend on the person in question (the risk factor may produce an adverse outcome in person A but not in person B); some risk factors are modifiable and can be mitigated by interventions. The existing literature is limited in providing us with precise, definitive, and generalizable information to assess these potential risks. Furthermore, perception of risk may be different from actual risk. The differing perception of risk can influence how prescribers present information to a patient, and how patients assimilate the information presented.

The process of choosing between treatment alternatives requires an assessment, acknowledgement, tolerance, and communication of the inherent uncertainty of the choices. Although empirical studies can inform estimates of treatment outcomes in certain situations, the generalizability and applicability of such data have limitations. For instance, the rate of relapse in the first year following the discontinuation of an antipsychotic medication in a patient with chronic schizophrenia has been reported as significantly higher than if the medication is continued (Leucht et al., 2009; Leucht et al., 2012). However, relapse rates are not 100% and we do not yet know how to confidently differentiate between patients who might relapse without medications and those who might not. Furthermore, we have limited confidence around what factors (besides medications) may impact the risk of relapse.

Creating a Constructive Environment

Ideally, decision-making is conducted in an environment where both patient and prescriber feel comfortable expressing their thoughts, wishes, and fears; sharing all relevant information including values and preferences; and interacting to reach a creative, individualized, and workable plan. When a discussion is personal and multifaceted, it is important that the persons concerned are able to express their opinions freely, without fear of rejection or ridicule. Questions like "What would you like the medication to help you with?" or "What do you think about taking this medication?" or "What about this medication makes you nervous?" may encourage patients to talk more in depth about their assumptions and experiences around taking medications. A plan of action arising from such a discussion will enlist the increased commitment of both prescriber and patient and may lead to a better outcome than a unilateral decision on either the patient's or the prescriber's part.

There are situations where the prescriber may agree to prescribe a medication that is not medically indicated largely because the patient's demands for it are perceived as unrelenting. Prescribers may want to avoid confrontation and increase trust, making it easier at times to prescribe what is not going to be a helpful medication but is one that will satisfy the patient (Brett & McCullough, 2012). A study measuring the effects of patient and prescriber expectations on prescribing behavior found that patients were more likely to receive a medication when the practitioner judged the patient to want the medication than when the practitioner ascribed no expectation to the patient (Cockburn & Pit, 1997). One way to address the effect of expectations on prescribing is to solicit them at the very beginning and clarify what medications can and cannot do.

Table 2.1 notes some of the important basic facets of creating an environment conducive to having initial discussions around the possibility of deprescribing medications.

Table 2.1 Creating an environment conducive to shared decision-making regarding deprescribing of medications

---

Timing
   If the symptom or problem being treated is not acute, take time before deciding whether or not to lower or stop medications, including adding psychosocial interventions if indicated

Attention
   Avoid answering the phone or using the computer (unless sharing information with the patient) during the appointment
   Frame a time and quiet setting dedicated to the conversation

Communication
   Use the "talk back" method to assess for understanding (Karen & Alan, 2017)
   Avoid discrediting or ridiculing patient sources
   Avoid interrupting the patient
   Ask questions to indicate that the patient is an equal partner in this decision ("What do you think?" "Do you have any suggestions about this?")

Effects and side effects
   Inquire actively about concerns about side effects, including sexual side effects
   Ask what the patient hopes the medication reduction will do

Attitude and approach
Be flexible. Emphasize that medication decisions are not a "one size fits all."
   Emphasize that the decision about medications is not binding and the medication can always be changed, adjusted or restarted
   If the patient prefers it, include friends or family in the discussion
   Tailor your approach to the patient. Patients expect and prefer varying degrees of involvement from their doctors. Even the same patient may want a different approach from their doctor at different points in their life

---

Evidence for Shared Decision-Making in Psychiatry

While there is strong evidence for SDM approaches improving certain outcomes and that it is desired by both patients and prescribers it is not yet ubiquitous (Davidson, Tondora, Pavlo & Stanhope, 2017). Certain concerns on the part of providers and psychiatrists may contribute to this, such as that, if left up to the patient, the decision will be a bad one (Beitinger et al., 2014; Hamann & Heres, 2014). In addressing this, the authors offer an outline to differentiate between different kinds of decisions that might call for a modified version of SDM, in particular issues more commonly faced by people with serious mental illness (see Figure 2.5).

The figure points to the differential decision-making approach depending on the type of decision. Deprescribing generally would fall into "best-choice" or "preference-sensitive" categories. At times deprescribing is actually the "best-choice" option but the patient still declines, with reasons including fear of relapse or other psychological factors discussed further in Chapters 3 and 4. Approaching these situations with care and utilizing methods like motivational interviewing or other approaches can slowly move a patient in the direction of considering a trial of deprescribing.

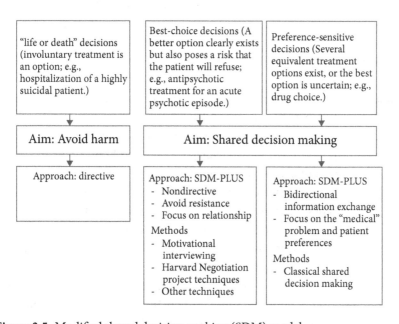

Figure 2.5 Modified shared decision-making (SDM) model.
From Hamann & Heres (2014). Reprinted with permission from the Psychiatric Services. American Psychiatric Association. All Rights Reserved.

Especially when the risks of polypharmacy are clear, a slow and careful discussion over a longer period of time (months or even years) is the indicated approach from our experience.

In psychiatry, and different from other specialities of medicine, it is important to keep in mind the extreme power differential represented by the power of the system to involuntarily commit someone. A patient's previous traumatic experiences with the mental health system may make having a real collaboration much more challenging.

Use of Language Around Medication

The movement toward recovery-oriented care and SDM is also reflected in the evolution of the terminology used to describe the degree of a patient's agreement and participation in the treatment. Accordingly, the terms used have changed from "compliance" to "adherence" and, more recently, "concordance" (Gutheil, 1982). *Compliance* is the extent to which a person's behavior (in terms of taking medications, following diets, or executing lifestyle changes) coincides with medical or health advice (Haynes et al., 1979). At times, courts and providers in mental health have used coercion to promote compliance, including such measures as involuntary hospitalization or outpatient treatment, threats of withholding resources (such as money), or lack of full disclosure of options or side effects (Corrigan, Kosyluk, & Kottsieper, 2015). *Adherence* is often used interchangeably with compliance but it is considered to be a more multidimensional phenomenon, one that may be influenced by patient- and health care provider–related factors, the therapy itself, education, and socioeconomic aspects. In some nonpsychiatric settings *adherence* is defined as filling prescriptions on time and *compliance* as taking medications as prescribed (Aronson, 2007). Generally, in mental health, the terms have both been used to describe taking medications as prescribed. "Persistence" is another term that is commonly used in time-limited fixed medication therapies such as cancer chemotherapy, although it has not been adopted in mental health (Andrade, Kahler, Frech, & Chan, 2006).

In psychiatry, the recovery model has suggested moving away from the word "compliance" because it implies that the patient is passive and unengaged. The more recent term in vogue, "adherence," has been used as a relatively less value-laden term with greater empowerment and active involvement of the patient. Most recently, the term "concordance" has been suggested as a less power-driven term and to represent the collaboration between prescriber and patient, although others have criticized the term as not capturing the patient behavior of following through with a prescribed course of medications (Aronson, 2007; Osterberge & Blaschke, 2005; Jordan, Ellis & Chambers, 2002).

In this book, we made the decision to use the term *adherence* because it describes the behavior of following a prescription made by the provider; although we agree that the term could be accused of not fully capturing the patient's participation in decision-making or the active nature of taking a medication as a means for desired life outcomes. The assumption is that the prescribed plan of care was a result of appropriate SDM.

A model for the continuum of decision-making from paternalism to collaboration is illustrated in Figure 2.6.

Some Additional Considerations

An important caveat in discussing a collaborative or shared decision-making model is that patients must retain the choice to *have the decision made by the prescriber*. Many patients, or even the same patient at different points in time, may prefer less information, less choice, and to rely on the prescriber's expertise without the burden of making the decision on their

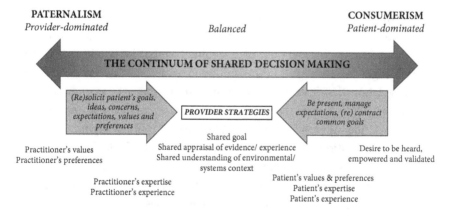

Figure 2.6 The continuum of decision-making in the prescriber–patient interaction.

own. This may seem contradictory to the idea of empowerment and choice, but it is an expression of choice in another way; to give up that choice and defer to another. The desire to have the prescriber be the decision-maker may also be culturally linked, where being able to rely on the prescriber to make the decision increases the comfort level of the patient. In more collectivist cultures, it may be essential and even the basic expectation for the family to be involved or for the parents of an adult child to make the decision for the child.

Regardless of one's personal feelings about the importance of patient involvement and collaboration, the decision to not make a decision is a valid one that also needs to be respected (Tondora et al., 2014). An insistence on the patient being "in the driver's seat" and making independent decisions in the name of person-centered care when that is not the preference of the person actually ends up contradicting these values instead of upholding them and errs toward *forced consumerism*. At the same time, it is essential to consider the previous messages and experiences that the person has been privy to within the mental health system. There may be significant learned helplessness and passivity within the "sick role." These attitudes may take time to shift and be unlearned, and they may appear to be the true "choice" of the person, but, with a bit of investigation and discussion, it can become clear that these choices are limited by the perceived expectations of the provider and the system.

Case Example

Cindy, a 57-year-old woman with a long history of schizophrenia, comes to the mental health center often. She has expressed occasional interest in reducing the dose of clozapine (she has been taking 500 mg each night for the past 8 years with good symptomatic control) due to the sedation that it causes. She would like to return to work and feels that she will likely fall asleep on the job with her current regimen. When the prescriber approaches her about potentially trying a slight reduction in her medications to address the fatigue, she says, "I don't know Doc, I've always been told staying on the meds is the most important thing. I probably shouldn't work anyway, it might stress me out even more. And I remember at the state hospital how many times they said I needed to reduce stress. So maybe it doesn't make sense for me to have a job. But I'll let you decide that, Doc."

Here it becomes clear that while the patient has a goal in mind—to get a job—she is conflicted due to messages she has received for many, many years about her vulnerability to stress. Cindy is reluctant to some extent to change anything about her medications due to the many years of messages regarding the importance of staying on them consistently and the metaphor ingrained in her—comparing the chronic management and prognosis of her mental illness to that of diabetes (which, as it was for her mother, she perceives to be progressive and incurable).

One way to handle this sometimes implicit or unconscious bias toward continuing medications unchanged is by asking questions such as, "What is the role of the medication in preventing a relapse *for this particular patient*? Does this patient place an equally high value on preventing relapse? What constitutes a relapse for this individual patient, and what else might prevent this? What else matters to the patient, and what are his or her preferences?" A summary of some possible questions as well as the associated framework is shown in Table 2.2.

Table 2.2 Questions that might help uncover and address the bias toward continuing medications unquestioned

Question	*Framework*
What is the role of this medication in preventing the relapse and/or treating symptoms?	Biopsychosocial perspective on relapse prevention
Does the patient value relapse prevention as much as I do?	Patient life goals and preferences
What does it mean to the patient to continue to be on medications?	Patient life goals and preferences
To what extent do these medications reduce risk?	Evidence for risk prevention (violence and self-harm, violence to others)
What does it mean to provide treatment in a situation where none might be needed?	The value of empirical evidence in treating the individual patient
What is the strength of the evidence that ongoing treatment is needed?	Critically evaluating existing evidence
What are the risks associated with continued medication treatment (and the benefits of potentially discontinuing)?	Risk–benefit analysis

Investigating potential implicit and explicit assumptions and beliefs around medication reduction may not change the ultimate course of action, but can be useful in decision-making. This is especially relevant when external factors (e.g., systemic pressures, family disagreement, fear of reprisal, fear of patient relapse, and liability issues) may ultimately be in conflict with patient preference and clinical judgment.

The Decision-Makers

The Prescriber as Expert

The prescriber is considered the expert on medical knowledge and is expected to make well-intentioned and informed treatment recommendations to the patient by integrating scientific knowledge and clinical experience. However, the prescriber's thinking process is not free of influences, internal and external, as well as conscious and unconscious. Prescribers unavoidably have their own values and preferences that affect their decisions and the parts of the evidence to which they pay attention. Different prescribers possess different abilities with respect to decision-making and integrating different kinds of information. A popular Oslerism calls medicine a science of uncertainty and an art of probability. Acknowledging and tolerating uncertainty is an important skill and essential to minimizing biases. An inability to acknowledge and tolerate uncertainty may cause us to ignore some therapeutic options, thereby allowing our biases to play a stronger role in our decision-making (Simpkin & Schwartzstein, 2016).

Often, providers may themselves find it difficult to assimilate outcomes of clinical studies expressed as complicated statistical parameters, much less communicate them effectively to a nervous and unwell patient. However, should the patient prefer, this information should be communicated in an understandable and effective way. For example, a study of women in cancer treatment found that they experienced less immediate satisfaction with the decision when the uncertainty of outcome was communicated clearly. The authors concluded that there was a tradeoff between the acknowledgment of uncertainty and decision satisfaction (Politi et al., 2011). The tradeoff may be well worth it if the final action is aligned with the patient's wishes, goals, and values after they have understood the available evidence for a course of action rather than a premature decision taken merely to allay anxiety as soon as possible.

The Patient as Expert

The patient is increasingly and perhaps controversially called an "expert by experience" or at a minimum, "an expert on their own experiences." This focus is to illustrate the importance of the person's perspective, as well as to serve as an empowering stance to decrease the power differential inherent in the prescriber–patient relationship (Gabbard & Nadelson, 1995). The patient brings an intimate knowledge of the conditions of their symptoms, the specific manifestations of such in the context of their daily life, and the goals and values that are important and have an impact in their decision-making process. This intersecting matrix of experience, goals, and values results in a unique configuration for each individual of how treatment would best suit the situation. Without full exploration and comfort in sharing these factors with the prescriber in a forthright way, the decision-making process may collapse from lack of clear understanding of an important factor or factors. Creating a trusting environment and a strong working alliance is therefore essential.

Conclusion

Decision-making in psychiatry is a complex process that is influenced by systemic and individual factors, both within the patient and the provider. Decision analysis consists of stages of *defining the problem, identifying alternatives, and choosing between them*, while SDM extends the more traditional medical approach to be a collaborative endeavor between prescriber and patient. Looking closely at the process of decision-making may help us identify our unconscious biases toward one course of action thereby encouraging evidence-based practice. Some common sources of biases in prescribers might be past experience; preferences of colleagues, mentors, and the institution at which one practices; advertising; and personal experiences. Viewing the deprescribing process as an opportunity to collaborate around an endeavor that can improve quality of life, physical health, and well-being means communicating clearly about preferences and values and taking time to planfully engage the patient in the process.

Self-Assessment

1. Alex is a 25-year-old man who dropped out of college 5 years ago because of a first episode of psychosis. He responded very well to risperidone long-acting injectable 50 mg every 2 weeks that was started within 3 weeks of his diagnosis. Three years ago, he dropped out of treatment for 4 months but returned when he started experiencing severe insomnia and anxiety again. He was restarted on the same medication and responded well to it again. Today, he is here to ask you about stopping the medication. He says that he doesn't feel like he is "normal" if he has to take medications to stay well. He also wants to go back to college and does not think that he can study while he is taking medication because it slows him down and makes his hands shake.
    a. What are the treatment options you would consider in this scenario?
    b. What are the treatment options you will offer Alex?
    c. If Alex asks you "what do you think would be best, doctor?" what would you say and why?
    d. What would your concerns be if you discontinued Alex's medications?
    e. What would your concerns be if you continued Alex's medications?
    f. Identify the source of these concerns and group them:
        i. Scientific literature
        ii. Past experience with similar patients
        iii. Intuition

2. Angela is a 35-year-old woman working as a teacher. She lives with her husband and her son who is 6 years old. She had a first episode of moderate major depression last year that responded well to sertraline 200 mg, and she has continued taking it for the past 18 months. She is thinking about having another child but is nervous about getting depressed again and does not want to stop the sertraline.

a. What are the treatment options you would consider in this scenario?
b. What are the treatment options you will offer Angela?
c. If Angela asks you "what do you think would be best doctor?" what would you say and why?
d. What would your concerns be if you discontinued Angela's medications?
e. What would your concerns be if you continued Angela's medications?
f. Identify the source of these concerns and group them:
   i. Scientific literature
   ii. Past experience with similar patients
   iii. Intuition

3. **Stages of shared decision-making include:**
   a. Choice talk, options talk, decision talk
   b. Assessment, alignment, agreement
   c. Explanation, discussion, decision
   d. Sharing, conflating, consensus

4. **A prescriber and patient meet, and the patient says, "Doc, please, don't tell me more, just tell me what to do." The treater, after some further discussion of the request, offers no further information to support the patient's decision-making and makes a recommendation. This is:**
   e. Authoritarianism
   f. Consistent with a person-centered approach
   g. Typical paternalism that is destructive to a collaboration
   h. A culturally insensitive approach

References

Adams, J. R., & Drake, R. E. (2006). Shared decision-making and evidence-based practice. *Community Mental Health Journal, 42*(1), 87–105.

Adams, N., & Grieder, D. M. (2004). *Treatment Planning for Person-Centered Care: The Road to Mental Health and Addiction Recovery.* New York: Elsevier Academic Press.

Andrade, S. E., Kahler, K. H., Frech, F., & Chan, K. A. (2006). Methods for evaluation of medication adherence and persistence using automated databases. *Pharmacoepidemiology and Drug Safety*, *15*(8), 565–574.

Aronson, J. K. (2007). Compliance, concordance, adherence. *British Journal of Clinical Pharmacology*, *63*(4), 383–384.

Beitinger, R., Kissling, W., & Hamann, J. (2014). Trends and perspectives of shared decision-making in schizophrenia and related disorders. *Current Opinions in Psychiatry*, *27*(3), 222–229. doi: 10.1097/yco.0000000000000057.

Brett, A. S., & McCullough, L. B. (2012). Addressing requests by patients for nonbeneficial interventions. *JAMA*, *307*(2), 149–150. doi: 10.1001/jama.2011.1999.

Brunette, M., Drake, R., & Lynde, D. (2002). *Integrated Dual Disorders Treatment Implementation Resource Kit*. Rockville, MD: Center for Mental Health Services, Substance Abuse and Mental Health Services Administration.

Cockburn, J., & Pit, S. (1997). Prescribing behaviour in clinical practice: Patients' expectations and doctors' perceptions of patients' expectations—a questionnaire study. *British Medical Journal*, *315*(7107), 520–523.

Collins, S. E., Carey, K. B., & Otto, J. M. (2009). A new decisional balance measure of motivation to change among at-risk college drinkers. *Psychology of Addictive Behaviors*, *23*(3), 464.

Corrigan, P. W., Kosyluk, K., & Kottsieper, P. (2015). The problem of adherence and the importance of self-determination. In P. Corrigan, ed. *Person-Centered Care for Mental Illness: The Evolution of Adherence and Self-Determination*. APA: Washington, DC, pp. 1–27.

Coylewright, M., Montori, V., & Ting, H. H. (2012). Patient-centered shared decision-making: A public imperative. *The American Journal of Medicine*, *125*(6), 545–547. doi: https://doi.org/10.1016/j.amjmed.2011.12.007.

Davidson, L., Tondora, J., Pavlo, A. J., & Stanhope, V. (2017). Shared decision-making within the context of recovery-oriented care. *Mental Health Review Journal*, *22*(3), 179–190.

Edwards, A., & Elwyn, G. (2009). *Shared Decision-Making in Health Care: Achieving Evidence-Based Patient Choice*. New York: Oxford University Press.

Elwyn, G., Frosch, D., Thomson, R., Joseph-Williams, N., Lloyd, A., Kinnersley, P., . . . Rollnick, S. (2012). Shared decision-making: A model for clinical practice. *Journal of General Internal Medicine*, *27*(10), 1361–1367.

Faraone, S. (1982). Psychiatry and political repression in the Soviet Union. *American Psychologist*, *37*(10), 1105.

Gabbard, G. O., & Nadelson, C. (1995). Professional boundaries in the physician-patient relationship. *JAMA*, *273*(18), 1445–1449.

Hamann, J., & Heres, S. (2014). Adapting shared decision-making for individuals with severe mental illness. *Psychiatric Services, 65*(12), 1483–1486.

Hamann, J., Leucht, S., & Kissling, W. (2003). Shared decision-making in psychiatry. *Acta Psychiatrica Scandinavica, 107*(6), 403–409.

Haynes, R. B., Taylor, D. W., & Sackett, D. L. (1979). *Compliance in health care.* Johns Hopkins University Press: Baltimore, US.

Janis, I. L., & Mann, L. (1977). *Decision-Making: A Psychological Analysis of Conflict, Choice, and Commitment.* New York: Free Press.

Jordan, J. L., Ellis, S. J., & Chambers, R. (2002). Defining shared decision-making and concordance: Are they one and the same? *Postgraduate Medical Journal, 78*(921), 383–384. doi: 10.1136/pmj.78.921.383.

Karen, J., & Alan, Q. (2017). The rationale for shared decision-making in mental health care; a systematic review of academic discourse. *Mental Health Review Journal, 22*(2), 152–165. doi: 10.1108/MHRJ-01-2017-0009.

Leucht, S., Arbter, D., Engel, R. R., Kissling, W., & Davis, J. M. (2009). How effective are second-generation antipsychotic drugs? A meta-analysis of placebo-controlled trials. *Molecular Psychiatry, 14*(4), 429–447.

Leucht, S., Tardy, M., Komossa, K., Heres, S., Kissling, W., Salanti, G., & Davis, J. M. (2012). Antipsychotic drugs versus placebo for relapse prevention in schizophrenia: A systematic review and meta-analysis. *The Lancet, 379*(9831), 2063–2071.

Mt-Isa, S., Hallgreen, C. E., Wang, N., Callréus, T., Genov, G., Hirsch, I., . . . Phillips, L. D. (2014). Balancing benefit and risk of medicines: A systematic review and classification of available methodologies. *Pharmacoepidemiology and Drug Safety, 23*(7), 667–678.

Osterberg, L., & Blaschke, T. (2005). Adherence to medication. *New England Journal of Medicine, 353*(5), 487–497.

Politi, M. C., Clark, M. A., Ombao, H., Dizon, D., & Elwyn, G. (2011). Communicating uncertainty can lead to less decision satisfaction: A necessary cost of involving patients in shared decision-making? *Health Expectations, 14*(1), 84–91.

Shippee, N. D., Shah, N. D., May, C. R., Mair, F. S., & Montori, V. M. (2012). Cumulative complexity: A functional, patient-centered model of patient complexity can improve research and practice. *Journal of Clinical Epidemiology, 65*(10), 1041–1051. doi: 10.1016/j.jclinepi.2012.05.005.

Simpkin, A. L., & Schwartzstein, R. M. (2016). Tolerating uncertainty—the next medical revolution? *New England Journal of Medicine, 375*(18), 1713–1715.

Strull, W. M., Lo, B., & Charles, G. (1984). Do patients want to participate in medical decision-making? *JAMA, 252*(21), 2990–2994. doi: 10.1001/jama.1984.03350210038026.

Tavakoli, M., Davies, H. T. O., & Thomson, R. (2000). Decision analysis in evidence-based decision-making. *Journal of Evaluation in Clinical Practice, 6*(2), 111–120.

Tondora, J., Miller, R., Slade, M., & Davidson, L. (2014). *Partnering for Recovery in Mental Health: A Practical Guide to Person-Centered Planning.* New York: John Wiley & Sons.

Wilson, S. R., Strub, P., Buist, A. S., Knowles, S. B., Lavori, P. W., Lapidus, J., & Vollmer, W. M. (2010). Shared treatment decision-making improves adherence and outcomes in poorly controlled asthma. *American Journal of Respiratory and Critical Care Medicine, 181*(6), 566–577.

3

Barriers to Deprescribing

Origins and Solutions

The goal of this chapter is to assist the reader in identifying potential barriers and solutions to the process of deprescribing. Deprescribing has the potential to streamline medication regimens, minimize side effects, and cut costs; the process also intends to improve patient adherence and strengthen the relationship between the patient and the prescribing professional. However, the patient–prescriber team may encounter numerous barriers while attempting this endeavor. Barriers may originate from the patient, prescriber, and/or the institution, both local and the larger medical system. This chapter frames potential general barriers and proposes ways to address them, with the caveat that any given prescriber–patient team may encounter context-specific barriers which need to be explored and addressed on a case-by-case basis.

Goal and Learning Objectives

After reading this chapter, the reader will be able to:

1. Recognize three prescriber-related factors that might bias against recommending deprescribing in any given scenario
2. Identify three barriers stemming from the patient and their environment that may be encountered when implementing deprescribing
3. Consider strategies for overcoming these barriers

Potential Pitfalls of Deprescribing

Risk of Relapse

In discussing deprescribing, one of the biggest fears for providers, patients, and family alike is that symptoms will reoccur in such a way to affect quality of life and/or functioning. In a relapsing/remitting illness (as many psychiatric conditions are regarded), there are specific clinical definitions. *Relapse* is a return to full syndrome once remission has occurred and *recurrence* is a further episode occurring after recovery as clinically defined across medical conditions. These have qualifications and thresholds based on the diagnostic criteria of the condition in question, and this will be discussed in more detail in each related chapter. Yet, between clinicians and among people with lived experience of mental illness, these terms are not commonly defined nor understood and often conflated as a single, colloquial construct of "relapse."

In other medical conditions, such as heart disease, another heart attack can be clearly delineated as a relapse of the underlying coronary disease. In mental health however, experiences considered to be a relapse by the patient can be quite individualized. For those who experience ongoing voices for example, and who consider those voices as symptoms, a relapse might be more usefully defined as an increased difficulty *coping* with voices (and subsequent hindering of work performance, for example) than an increase in the frequency of the voices themselves. The functional impairment that results from an increase in symptoms may be more relevant than an actual increase in and of itself. The relative difference and degree of difference from one psychological state to the next is important in this more personalized definition of relapse and may be conjointly agreed upon by prescriber and client in discussions surrounding deprescribing.

The outcome of hospitalization has been widely used as a marker of relapse in mental health research. Alternatively, Lader identifies two other general categories: a change in severity of psychopathology and a deterioration in social functioning or social roles. A majority of published studies in schizophrenia use hospitalization to define relapse, over clinical scales such as the PANSS and CGI (see Olivares et al., 2013 for a review). Hospitalization represents a heterogeneous set of factors and may not capture the experiences of people who might have an exacerbation of symptoms without hospitalization or may be hospitalized strategically for a medication adjustment (which, in their experience, does not rise to the definition of relapse *per se*). In other words, relapse is not a one-size-fits-all concept, can be individually defined by the person, and may or may not denote an increase in symptoms.

We should be under no illusion - it is well-documented that discontinuation of psychotropic agents increases the risk of relapse in recurrent depressive disorder, bipolar disorder, and schizophrenia. The caveats are that discontinuation studies in all three disorders have methodological limitations (as discussed in further chapters), and crucially, we argue that *discontinuation* (as is has been variably implemented thus far in psychiatric research) *is not an equivalent intervention to deprescribing*. Instead, deprescribing is a holistic intervention looking at the *possibility* of reducing or stopping medication while engaging in extensive preplanning, prevention, and possibly the addition of other interventions and supports. Nonetheless, the risks of deprescribing must be discussed clearly with the patient to the extent that those risks can be assessed. Factors to consider include experiences of past attempts at medication reduction, current substance use, psychosocial stressors, and levels of support. Although for some people relapses and rehospitalizations can be disruptive to employment, relationships, and stable housing, it may be important to consider that a patient may choose to risk a relapse or rehospitalization rather than continuing to take a medication that presents for them a more insidious and chronic biological (e.g., side effects), psychological (e.g., meaning of the medication or impact on self-efficacy), or social (e.g., cost or stigma) burden.

Deprescribing and Stigmatization of Mental Illness and Its Treatment

One of our goals in arguing for deprescribing in psychiatry is to promote individualized medication treatments at minimum effective doses integrated into a multi-dimensional care plan, thus promoting and furthering the idea of using medication as one of many tools in the recovery process. If deprescribing is applied indiscriminately and is viewed as endorsing "antipsychiatry" perspectives, then such application will defeat our fundamental purpose of maximizing the benefits of medication while minimizing harm in order to promote better quality of life for each individual, considering his or her unique set of circumstances. If deprescribing is misinterpreted or misused, it could also serve to reinforce the stigma associated with appropriate treatments for psychiatric disorders. The intent of deprescribing is not to demonize the use of medications, nor to send a message that medication use is problematic. Many people with mental illness describe wanting to discontinue their medications because this will somehow prove that they are 'well' or that they don't have mental illness after all (see Roe, Goldblatt, Baloush-Klienman, Swarbrick, & Davidson, 2008). While the approach of deprescribing is value-neutral on these ideas and does not take a universal stance regarding the meaning of medications, it is essential to consider these feelings and associations in the process of deprescribing in order to best support the intervention on an individual, a systems, and a societal level (see Chapter 4 for further discussion).

Physician-Related Factors

Large surveys conducted among geriatricians and primary care physicians identified the following barriers to deprescribing: uncertainty over why drugs were prescribed in the first place, concern over an increased workload (including the time required), and a fear of not following accepted guidelines and the potential consequences of such, including but not limited to litigation (see Reeve et al., 2013). We suggest that these, as well as other reasons, can readily arise in the practice of deprescribing as applied to psychiatry.

The lack of a clearly identified purpose by the original prescriber of the medication can introduce doubt and concern for the current prescriber (e.g., "Is there something another provider saw that I am missing? Has the patient underreported their symptoms and there is a compelling reason for this prescription after all? What negative consequence might there be if the medication is reduced or discontinued?"). These doubts and uncertainties can result in faltering, if not wholly rejected, attempts at deprescribing.

It is important to reflect on what stops prescribers from considering the option of medication reduction despite the standard guidelines recommending the use of minimum effective doses (as described in Table 3.1). Physicians, in general, have been reported to be perfectionistic, harm-avoidant, and risk-averse (Eley, Young, & Przybeck, 2009; Kluger, Laidlaw, Kruger, & Harrison, 1999). Reduction or discontinuation of medications

Table 3.1 Reasons why prescribers might hesitate to consider medication reduction or discontinuation when a patient is well

Reasoning	Cultural, personal, or professional value attached to this reasoning
• Symptoms may reappear if medication is reduced	• We want to reduce suffering, not increase it
• The patient may relapse if medication is reduced	• Understanding relapse as failure of treatment and we don't want to fail
• Absence of *guidelines* for medication reduction	• We don't want to do what we haven't been trained to do; nobody has taught us how to do it
• Absence of *indications* for medication reduction	• There's no immediately apparent reason to do it; nobody has told us to do it
• Minimize risk to the patient and society	• Prescribing is less risky than deprescribing, continuation of medications is the most efficient way to minimize risk, sociocultural incentivization of medication prescribing over deprescribing
• The patient may relapse if medication is reduced	• Avoiding blame/litigation for a relapse
• Psychiatric diagnoses are lifetime diagnoses	• Professional training highlights this statement as a fact

may mean increasing the risk of symptoms, relapse, or even the need to hospitalize a patient—a result that is often viewed as a failure by the prescriber and the system. The drive to prevent a relapse can be so strong that medication reduction and/or discontinuation might not occur to a prescriber, missing an opportunity for improvement of quality of life for the patient. Furthermore, managed care limits the time afforded to the prescriber and the patient to adequately devote to the process of shared decision-making, and continuing medications unchanged is thus incentivized as a 'safe' default.

"If It Ain't Broke, Don't Fix It"

Nonmaleficence is a deeply rooted ethical principle in medicine, but when unbalanced by other principles, could validate unnecessary, prolonged medication regimens. Indeed, errors of *omission* may seem more forgivable than errors of *commission*. Framing this sentiment more emphatically is the phrase "never change a winning team," which evokes a metaphor to imply that victory serves as an indicator that a particular combination of players (or medications) functions optimally and indefinitely (Nüesch & Haas, 2012). While 'never changing the winning team' may be a compelling approach for a college football coach for the season, over the years, as the average age of the team approaches 90 (let us say), lesser success may be enjoyed. A similar distinction may be applied to prescribing, where what works initially may not necessarily bear out through the entire natural course, or indeed life of the patient. Complicating factors might include normal aging, co-occuring medical conditions, psychosocial conditions, and stakeholder preference. For instance, infectious disease consultants have reported that many primary treatment teams tend to prefer continuing the original antibiotic therapy if they have obtained desirable results, despite specialist recommendations for a streamlining of antibiotic therapy (Van der Meer & Gyssens, 2001).

Overapplication of this rubric can manifest in many different ways in psychiatric prescribing, for example (1) in extended treatment with anticholinergics in the absence of proven risk of antipsychotic-induced extrapyramidal symptoms (Marsden & Jenner, 1980); (2) in persistence with higher doses of antipsychotic medications (where lower dose antipsychotic treatment can be a viable option in the maintenance phase; Schooler, 1993, 1991); and (3) in the continuation of polypharmacy without establishing each individual medications' ongoing need (Stahl & Grady, 2004). That being said, Onder, Nobili, and Margenoni (2016) add a cautionary note about disparaging this ethical principle and excessive enthusiasm for deprescribing in geriatrics where, in complex patients, medical stability may be precarious and hard-won after several combinations have been already tried. This argument, too, can be easily applied to psychiatry where rational polypharmacy (e.g. antidepressant augmentation and specific combinations of mood stabilizers and antipsychotics) has a steadily growing evidence base.

What To Do About It

It behooves the prescriber to remember that the decision to continue a medication regimen unchanged remains a decision made. Ethical practice and sound clinical decision-making demand representation from and weighing of multiple perspectives. A prescriber must remain mindful of whether one's practice could be biased in one direction or another (i.e., more prone in general to suggest a change or promote continuation relative to peers). The simplest and most acceptable approach to challenging blinkered nonmaleficence is the use of credible evidence from sources such as national guidelines that, for example, recommend the active seeking of minimal effective doses as standard practice. It might also be worthwhile to remind ourselves that, in addition to allaying symptoms at the current time, we bear the responsibility of minimizing the potential for serious side effects that may occur in the future. The latter involves maintaining a balance between an active treatment approach and a preventive approach in the management of medications. For instance, it is known that the incidence of antipsychotic-induced tardive dyskinesia increases with age and the duration of antipsychotic treatment. Similarly, the rate of lithium-induced permanent tubule-interstitial renal disease has been reported to increase with the duration of treatment. Remaining mindful of the accumulating risk of these serious side effects while renewing these medications may help in overcoming any fears regarding considering a deprescribing process and thus "rocking the boat."

Limited Guidelines on Deprescribing

Training and guidelines in psychopharmacology are largely focused on the initiation, continuation, and monitoring of medication treatment and do not equally describe the process of medication withdrawal and/or discontinuation, which are typically only mentioned in the context of switching from one psychotropic to another (i.e. cross-titration). For instance, standard guidelines for the management of depression address the use of "washout" and cross-tapering when switching from one antidepressant to another but offer relatively fewer suggestions for when a patient may want to collaborate around stopping an antidepressant drug and not replace it with another. Guidelines for management of schizophrenia recommend the use of minimum effective doses of antipsychotics in the maintenance phase of treatment but do not outline a tapering schedule or what to do when a patient wishes to collaboratively try a medication-free period. In these situations, a novice prescriber, by virtue of their training experiences, may be disincentivized towards change. Until more formal training and guidelines exist, prescribers might reassure themselves that their training offers relevant and translatable knowledge and skills. To further provide perspective (although not yet formally studied, but drawing on universally-reported high rates of non-adherence) one might posit that the majority of medication tapers and discontinuations undertaken are in fact instigated and 'managed' by patients alone.

What To Do About It

Lack of current guidelines around deprescribing requires the prescriber to take a more creative and innovative approach. Gaining comfort with this experience may necessitate additional peer and team support for the prescriber. Providers might draw on the past experiences of the patients themselves, as patients are likely to have had past experiences with discontinuing medications without informing their prescribers. Hence persons with relevant lived experience may be considered a valuable partner. As the literature addressing optimal medication withdrawal strategies still grows, persons with lived experience of self-managed discontinuations, perhaps guided by online resources such as consumer forums, may arguably hold the majority of the collective expertise on the topic. Of course, utmost caution and scrutiny should be exercised when integrating anecdotal evidence (particularly from patient forums) into one's understanding. Beyond the limited published literature, discussions with more experienced colleagues can also prove to be an invaluable resource. The peer-reviewed publication of anecdotal evidence, such as case reports, can lay the foundations for the generation of higher levels of evidence. All readers are encouraged to contribute to this effort. Currently, there is a wealth of untapped clinical experience among colleagues, patients, and other care providers that can be informally tapped for potential guidance. By drawing on these various resources, the application of fundamental priniciples and listening to one's patient, the novice deprescriber can be better equipped and feel more confident in their approach to deprescribing.

Fear of a Bad Clinical Outcome and Potential Litigation

In a nationwide survey of barriers to deprescribing among psychiatrists, a fear of relapse and rehospitalization emerged as a central concern (Gupta, 2018). Given the mixed results of numerous observational as well as randomized controlled trials of medication discontinuation in patients with schizophrenia, bipolar disorder, and recurrent depression, and the subsequent guidelines that have emerged from these trials, this concern is more than valid. This fear is intensified when considering patients with past histories of suicide attempts, violence, and criminal justice system contact. Furthermore, an attempt at deprescribing may be perceived as flouting standard guidelines or not providing best common practice, leaving the prescriber potentially vulnerable to litigation.

What To Do About It

An awareness of the "therapeutic illusion" or the "illusion of control" may help mitigate the fear of relapse to some extent. The therapeutic illusion has been defined as a situation where physicians believe that their actions or tools are more effective than they actually are and is based on the tendency of human beings to overestimate the effect of their actions (Casarett, 2016; Langer, 1975; Thomas, 1978). This perpetuates the idea that withdrawal or change in a medication (as the more salient action) *will* destabilize a patient, which in turn causes the prescriber to keep the medication unchanged. Casarett (2016) recommends two questions to ask ourselves in helping to dispel or challenge our innate tendency toward the therapeutic illusion. First, "before you conclude that a treatment was effective, look for other explanations," and, second, "if you see evidence of success, look for evidence of failure." Applying these principles to psychiatry may reveal, for instance, that what we perceived as a good response to an antipsychotic was actually explained by the patient simultaneously securing disability benefits. This relates as well to the statistical adage "correlation does not equal causation," another useful maxim in potentially dispelling the illusion. One might accordingly also question why our patients who continue to accept their prescriptions unwaveringly still end up having relapses.

Patient-Related Factors

Reeve et al. (2013), in their review of 21 articles, identified three themes within the potential barriers to and enablers of deprescribing in older individuals. These were disagreement or agreement with "appropriateness" of cessation, absence or presence of a "process" for cessation, and negative or positive "influences" to the idea of ending the use of a particular medication (Reeve et al., 2013). Numerous other potential reasons prevent people from asking their physicians to reduce the number of medications.

Patients may fear a relapse of illness, fear being denied the ability to resume medication, or even fear provoking disapproval or abandonment by their treaters, especially if they have previously had negative reactions to the suggestion of decreasing medication. Avoidance of the issue may lead some patients to discontinue medications unilaterally—which may deprive the prescriber of the opportunity to collaborate and gain experience with this process.

Fear of Relapse

Patients have often worked hard to achieve symptom control with the right combination of medications. It is understandable that a person may be reluctant and even strongly opposed to any change in medications because of the fear of the return of symptoms or a concern about being rehospitalized. This fear may be reinforced by shared feelings in treaters, by institutionalizing attitudes that equate clinical status solely with medication adherence and by repeatedly-heard advice to stay on their medications in order to stay well.

At the same time, although a useful tool, the process of self-monitoring can have the unintended consequence of developing hypervigilance in the person with mental illness; a constant watching of the self for any emergence of symptoms. This can lead to anxiety regarding mood fluctuations, for example, that may be "within normal limits" or not really a concern. In this way the anxiety triggered by the fear of relapse can contribute to a self-fulfilling prophesy. Therefore, as Gumley puts it, there is a need to "de-catastrophize relapse" (Gumley & Schwannauer, 2006).

One useful scale for assessing fear of relapse is the Fear of Recurrence scale (FORSE; Gumley & Schwannauer, 2006), which assesses the concerns of a person regarding *recurrence* (used interchangeably with *relapse* in reference to this scale). The scale includes three subscales: fear of relapse, awareness of thoughts, and intrusiveness. This is based on research evidence that the appraisals and increase in focus and self-consciousness about experiences and bodily sensation actually contribute to the increase in distress and an acceleration of potential relapse (Gumley, White, & Power, 1999). The "fear of relapse" subscale had strong correlations with anxiety and depression further supporting the idea that concerns about relapse may further speed symptom onset.

What To Do About It

Listening to and validating the patient's concerns about relapse may be the first step in addressing them. Of note, it may take months or even years to consolidate an alliance sufficiently secure for a patient to even consider changing a medication. The prescriber should strive to minimize unaddressed issues that might bias a collaborative weighing of the risk–benefit ratio for a medication. This might include proactively educating against the barriers outlined in this chapter as well as modeling acceptance of uncertainty. Development of a detailed plan to identify relapse or symptom return early on may be a useful step in reassuring the person about their ability to decrease medications in a safe, controlled way. For someone accustomed to being sedated and having their moods and distress muted, the return of intense emotional experiences may be both a delight and contain an element of terror, for fear that these experiences are the harbinger of a relapse. Expanding the definition of health by shrinking the idea and definitional boundaries of relapse may be useful in the process of deprescribing a medication. Normalizing variations in mood and experiences of distress can be seen as important targets in supporting a person to weather the potential of increased variation of experiences as the effect of medications are lessened.

Impact on Family, Friends, and Caregiver Relationships

Sometimes, the relationships that patients develop feel as if they may be (or are) contingent on the patient continuing to take medications. For instance, a spouse may have already threatened divorce unless medications are taken, or the patient may fear that friends will abandon a patient if they become symptomatic. Some relationships may have been initially forged around having a psychiatric treatment in common (e.g. meeting a friend at clozapine group). Treatment relationships (prescriber, therapist, clinician, case manager) as well as those stemming from treatment (e.g. friends met at the mental health center) can be significant, and a desire to please, or at least not risk disappointing a caregiver may discourage a patient from instigating a change in a prescribed treatment. Many patients are socially connected to their visiting nurse who administers medications; discontinuing medications might end these twice daily visits to their home. A patient may fear that deprescribing might mean less frequent contact with a prescriber to whom they are attached and from whom they have received significant support.

What To Do About It

If the patient feels comfortable and wishes to, the easiest way to address pressure from family, friends, or even wider treatment team members, is to engage them, at some stage, in the decision-making and implementation process of deprescribing. Involving significant social supports and allaying their anxiety may be as or more important as allaying the patient's anxiety. More specific interventions, such as couples therapy or family therapy, may be indicated. Deprescribing may be framed in a positive light, as a routine treatment option from the outset, without threat of diminishing or jeopardizing the therapeutic relationship. Patients may also feel as if their prescriber is abandoning them during deprescribing or even at the suggestion of deprescribing, making it essential to address these concerns immediately and even if they do not come up directly. One might frame the importance and utility of continuing (and even more frequent) periodic followup irrespective of prescribing. When it is the case, i.e. routine follow up with the psychiatrist will continue, it may be useful to explicitly state that this relationship, at least, is not contingent on taking medications.

Fear of Losing Benefits

It is commonly perceived that applications for benefits such as social security disability income (SSDI) and other services such as in-home care, individual or group therapy, or rehabilitation services are strengthened by listing medications in the application form. Indeed, the psychosocial interventions patients engage in to sustain their recovery can be more challenging to quantify and articulate. A long list of medications at high doses may paint an individual as being very ill and therefore highly deserving of disability benefits. Although perhaps not accurately reflecting the decision-making process of any adjudicating body, the potential role of medications as "badges of illness" may lead a patient to imagine that they are at risk of losing their benefits if their application is weakened by a diminished medication list.

What To Do About It

Effective and direct communication of the patient's clinical and functional status (including documentation of nonpharmaceutical strategies) with the concerned authority may be needed. Reasons for medication discontinuation (e.g., ineffectiveness or side effects) may have to be noted in the supporting documentation. While reassuring the patient directly may be tempting, it is important to temper this with the realistic possibility that benefits may be cut or lost, and that as the prescriber or clinician it is impossible to provide any true guarantee. Just as patients assume that a long list is supportive of more serious impairment, it is not clear that the assessors may not have similar assumptions. Providing detailed rationale and accurate current functioning, and being transparent with the patient about the framing and even sharing the document with the patient, can help reduce anxiety and support the alliance in the worst case scenario in which benefits are denied.

Withdrawal or Rebound Symptoms

Although medications such as benzodiazepines and opioids (causing tolerance and dependence) are most notable for their classic withdrawal syndromes, serotonergic antidepressants such as selective serotonin reuptake inhibitors (SSRIs), tricyclic antidepressants (TCAs) and serotonin and norepinephrine reuptake inhibitors (SNRIs) are also associated with clinically salient discontinuation (or withdrawal) syndromes. Furthermore, these serotonin withdrawal symptoms may resemble the underlying illness (mood lability, transient depression, severe anxiety), and both patient and prescriber may become concerned about a relapse. Patients may change their mind about deprescribing because of how difficult it can be to tolerate and manage these distressing, yet transient symptoms. Hopefully less relevant to a well-implemented deprescribing, abrupt discontinuation of other psychotropics (e.g. lithium and antipsychotics) have been linked to rebound symptoms resembling a recurrence of the underlying condition. Withdrawal syndromes are discussed in more detail in the relevant chapters that follow.

What To Do About It

Just as transient, 'initiation' side effects should be mentioned when prescribing a new medication, preparation for withdrawal symptoms while deprescribing is crucial. Preparation may involve creating expectations and providing information about the nature and potential duration of withdrawal symptoms, along with a plan of management. Reassurance that withdrawal symptoms can be effectively managed and are time-limited may be very helpful in averting the patient's conclusion that they have become forever reliant on the medication to feel well. A plan to manage rebound symptoms or recurrence may include close surveillance, a planned response and *apriori* acceptance of the possibility that it may become necessary to slow the taper or even retitrate to a higher dosage in order to regroup and reassess the deprescribing plan.

Deprescribing and Identity Disruption

Some individuals receiving long-term services within large, encompassing institutions such as the public mental health system become socialized into an identity of "being a patient." This identity is constructed around a core self-perception through the lens of psychiatric diagnosis and treatment. Withdrawal of medication, or even a suggestion thereof, could threaten a potential loss of identity. Patients may even have daily or weekly routines (yielding collateral benefits such as structured social contact) constructed around obtaining and filling prescriptions as well as taking the drugs themselves. These routines for many people include having developed strong social relationships with those care providers involved in medication administration. For example, a patient's brief daily interaction with their visiting nurse may represent their most significant social contact. Alternatively, a periodic visit to the friendly local pharmacy might prompt another patient to treat themselves to some new toiletries or self-care items each month. The idea of discontinuing medications may trigger both a loss of identity (whether it be socially valued or devalued) as well as the loss of corresponding everyday social interactions and ritual which are associated with accessing and administering the medication.

What To Do About It
Appropriate framing of the place of medications in treatment at the time of prescribing may help patients 'let go' of them when they are not needed anymore. A discussion on what it means for the person to be on a psychotropic medication can be a rich area for discovery of meaning and associations

that the person may not be fully aware of initially. Following this discussion, exploring what it might mean to lead a life without medications may be helpful. Exploration of the practical activities surrounding the regimen, collateral benefits, and what they stand to lose presents an opportunity to find alternatives to relationships mediated by medication tasks. Increasing other social supports can assist the person in thinking through deprescribing. The recovery literature has suggested that one of the challenges associated with recovery may be the task of accepting oneself as an ordinary agentic (having agency) human being, a task that may very well emerge during deprescribing as well.

Systemic and Cultural Factors

Association of Medication with Health Rather than Disease

With the commodification of health, supplements; screening tests; provider visits; and to some degree medications have come to be associated with health and maintenance of health rather than treatment of disease. Instead of assuming the baseline of a healthy body that does not require any medications, consumers may feel like they are missing out on health if they are not taking a certain number of medications. This can be problematic when this attitude disincetivizes more favorable wellness strategies (such as decreasing alcohol use, or getting more exercise). In such a societal climate, an intervention such deprescribing may be easily perceived as withdrawal of care or deprivation. Garfinkel (2017) stress that the concept of deprescribing may be automatically perceived as a negative approach, one interfering with "good health." For instance, in Ireland, when the health service incentivized the reduction of antibiotic prescriptions it was perceived by the public as inadequate care for patients (see Wise, 2016).

Pressure from Direct-to-Consumer Advertising

"Ask your doctor today, if drug x is right for you" is a commonly heard phrase on television. When patients are bombarded with commercials and printed advertisements eulogizing the benefits of a particular brand of medication, they may view the receipt of the free samples as a boon and subsequent discontinuation as deprivation. Direct-to-consumer advertising may influence prescribers to offer medications they may not have otherwise prescribed (due to relative appropriateness, confidence, or experience). In a recent survey, more than 33% of participants said that they asked their prescribers for information about a drug they had seen or heard advertised, and almost 25% asked for a prescription of that drug. Seventy-five percent of these individuals reported that their prescribers gave them the requested drug (American Pharmaceutical Association, 1997).

What To Do About It
At the time of writing, the United States is only one of two countries that allows direct-to-consumer advertising (the other being New Zealand—although this is under review as the medical community lobbies against potential detrimental effects). On the level of the individual patient–provider relationship, all sources of information can be acknowledged, contextualized and integrated. The appeal from marketing can be acknowledged and weighed within the risk–benefit calculation as either positive or negative. For some patients, a marketing campaign may bring value in the form of buy-in or alternatively create unrealistic expectations for results; checking in with the patient as to the source of their information can help clarify and contribute to a conversation that is forthright and respectful.

Time Constraints and Absence of Coordinated Systems of Care

Deprescribing is a time-intensive intervention requiring detailed review of the risks and benefits of each medication, coordination with other prescribers, and the development of a multidisciplinary plan for the prevention of relapse. In the age of '15-minute medication checks' (Torrey, Griesemer, & Carpenter-Song, 2017), most psychiatrists merely have sufficient time to review changes in symptoms and side effects, order refills, and complete the patient record. Support from pharmacists, primary care providers, and a good communication network are all essential for supporting effective deprescribing. Attempts at coordinating care with other prescribers may not always prove successful, especially in the absence of common electronic health record systems. When this infrastructure is unavailable, well-meaning prescribers who would otherwise support deprescribing may be feel daunted by the time investment required and feel compelled to abandon it as a nonessential or unfeasible intervention.

What To Do About It

Although cultures of practice can be gradually influenced, systemic barriers can warrant interventions at the level of the agency and institution, as well as looking at broader mental health and healthcare policy change. This might include advocacy at the state and federal levels. The specific issue of insufficient time for pursuing a deprescribing intervention may be addressed in at least two ways. At the systems level, in most instances it is the insurance carriers that influence the level of detail/complexity and/or duration of the physician–patient encounter through economic incentives and disincentives. One potential avenue for change in this area would be providing, via billing parameters, evidence for the overall long-term cost-effectiveness of deprescribing and creating a set of billing codes or bundled payment specific to this intervention. At the individual patient level, with limited available duration or frequency of visits, time costs may be defrayed longitudinally. Alternatively, a long-term therapeutic relationship with a prescriber can be leveraged. The strength of the therapeutic alliance may provide a safety net in a sense, allowing the patient to take more risks because of confidence in their relationship with the provider. Typically deprescribing is not something that needs to, or should, be rushed. Spreading the process over multiple meetings allows for intersession assignments for both patient and prescriber. Written information and other materials (such as specialized decision support tools) may be reviewed at a patient's leisure. The assumption that deprescribing requires a prohibitive amount of time and effort within our current systems of care should be countered.

Conclusion

Deprescribing can be challenging to implement due to factors stemming from prescribers, patients, caregivers, and the surrounding cultures and systems of care. Prescribers may be disinclined to deprescribe due to relative lack of time and/or training, concern of violating standard guidelines, and concerns of "causing" a relapse or risk-taking behavior (i.e., harm to self or others). Patients, on the other hand, may resist deprescribing due to a fear of symptom recurrence; pressure from family, friends, or mental health staff; and concern for other collateral consequences such as losing valued resources. Systemic and institutional factors such as a societal "pressure to prescribe" and brief medication management visits may further dissuade providers from altering the status quo. Barriers can be addressed through the better training of prescribers, both at the level of core and specialty training; ongoing education of patients about their medications; dynamic updating of the risk–benefit calculation; and further influencing public attitudes to health as a process and lifestyle and not an "off the shelf" commodity merely to be consumed.

Self-Assessment

1. Joe is 40-year-old single unemployed man receiving social security disability who lives with his elderly mother. He was diagnosed with schizoaffective disorder in his 20s and takes haloperidol 5 mg twice a day, olanzapine 30 mg at bedtime, and benztropine 2 mg in the morning (without which he experiences extrapyramidal side effects). Between the ages of 25 and 31 he had eight hospitalizations for threatening behavior toward his mother. You look at his medication regimen and wonder if he might still do well without the haloperidol. When you broach this question with Joe and his mother, they are immediately reluctant.

    a. How might you engender further discussion about attempting to deprescribe the haloperidol and what would be the indication?
    b. Speculate on three reasons which Joe might be declining a reduction in this medication.
    c. What kind of psycho-social interventions may support deprescribing in this case?

2. Mary is a 67-year-old woman who lives in a rest home. She was diagnosed as having schizophrenia in her 30s and has taken clozapine 200 mg twice a day for 15 years. She also has type 2 diabetes and hypertension and has suffered two strokes. You suggest a slow reduction in dose, to which she is amenable, but she struggles to relate back the rationale during your initial discussion. She is not conserved, but her family heavily influences her care at the home. That evening her nurse from the rest home calls, incredulous, wondering whether

what Mary is relating to her about today's appointment is true, "Her daughter will never allow this!"

    a. What are the potential risks of reducing Mary's dose?

    b. Speculate on three potential concerns that the nurse might have.

    c. How will you address the nurse's concerns regarding deprescribing?

3. **Tim is a 29-year-old man who has continued escitalopram following two major depressive episodes. He has been seeing you monthly since he had his first episode at age 23 and the second at 26. Both episodes were in the context of major life events. Although he believes the medication was helpful in remitting his depression, he is wondering whether he should stop the escitalopram, with his fiancée often telling him that "it is a sign of weakness."**

    a. What are the risks of engaging in a deprescribing of escitalopram?

    b. Speculate on three possible reasons driving Tim's ambivalence about stopping the medication.

    c. How might you overcome these barriers and proceed with a deprescribing?

References

American Pharmaceutical Association (1997). *Navigating the Medication Marketplace: HowConsumersChoose* (Washington: *Prevention*/American Pharmaceutical Association, 1997).

Casarett, D. (2016). The Science of Choosing Wisely—Overcoming the Therapeutic Illusion. *New England Journal of Medicine, 374*(13), 1203–1205. doi: 10.1056/NEJMp1516803

Eley, D., Young, L., & Przybeck, T. R. (2009). Exploring the temperament and character traits of rural and urban doctors. *The Journal of Rural Health, 25*(1), 43–49.

Garfinkel, D. (2017). Overview of current and future research and clinical directions for drug discontinuation: Psychological, traditional and professional obstacles to deprescribing. *European Journal of Hospital Pharmacology, 24*(1), 16–20.

Gumley, A., & Schwannauer, M. (2006). *Staying Well After Psychosis: A Cognitive Interpersonal Approach to Recovery and Relapse Prevention.* New York: John Wiley & Sons.

Gumley, A., White, C. A., & Power, K. (1999). An interacting cognitive subsystems model of relapse and the course of psychosis. *Clinical Psychology & Psychotherapy*, 6(4), 261–278. doi: doi:10.1002/(SICI)1099–0879(199910)6:4<261::AID-CPP211>3.0.CO;2-C.

Gupta, S., Miller, R., Montenegro, R., Pavlo, A., Cahill, J.,D. (2018). Survey of Practices, Attitudes and Barriers to Deprescribing Psychiatric Medications. *Poster presented at: Annual conference of the American Psychiatric Association, New York.*

Lader, M. (1995). What is relapse in schizophrenia? *International Clinical Psychopharmacology*, 9, 5–10.

Langer, E. J. (1975). The illusion of control. *Journal of personality and social psychology*, 32(2), 311.

Marsden, C., & Jenner, P. (1980). The pathophysiology of extrapyramidal side-effects of neuroleptic drugs. *Psychological Medicine*, 10(1), 55–72.

Nüesch, S., & Haas, H. (2012). Empirical evidence on the "Never Change a Winning Team" heuristic. *Jahrbücher für Nationalökonomie und Statistik*, 232(3), 247–257.

Olivares, J. M., Sermon, J., Hemels, M., & Schreiner, A. (2013). Definitions and drivers of relapse in patients with schizophrenia: A systematic literature review. *Annals of General Psychiatry*, 12(1), 32. doi: 10.1186/1744–859x-12–32.

Onder, G., Nobili, A., & Marengoni, A. (2016). Potentially inappropriate drug prescribing and the "never change a winning team" principle. *Journals of Gerontology Series A: Biomedical Sciences and Medical Sciences*, 71(11), 1531–1532.

Reeve, E., To, J., Hendrix, I., Shakib, S., Roberts, M. S., & Wiese, M. D. (2013). Patient barriers to and enablers of deprescribing: a systematic review. *Drugs & Aging*, 30(10), 793–807.

Roe, D., Goldblatt, H., Baloush-Klienman, V., Swarbrick, M., & Davidson, L. (2008). Why and how people decide to stop taking prescribed psychiatric medication: Exploring the subjective process of choice. *Psychiatric Rehabilitation Journal*, 33(1), 38–46.

Schooler, N. R. (1993). Reducing dosage in maintenance treatments of schizophrenia: Review and prognosis. *British Journal of Psychiatry Supplement*, 22, 58–65.

Schooler, N. R. (1991). Maintenance medication for schizophrenia: strategies for dose reduction. *Schizophrenia Bulletin*, 17(2), 311–324.

Stahl, S., & Grady, M. (2004). A critical review of atypical antipsychotic utilization: Comparing monotherapy with polypharmacy and augmentation. *Current Medicinal Chemistry*, 11(3), 313–327.

Thomas, K. (1978). The consultation and the therapeutic illusion. *British Medical Journal, 1*(6123), 1327–1328.

Torrey, W. C., Griesemer, I., & Carpenter-Song, E. A. (2017). Beyond "med management." *Psychiatric Services, 68*(6), 618–620.

Van der Meer, J., & Gyssens, I. (2001). Quality of antimicrobial drug prescription in hospital. *Clinical Microbiology and Infection, 7*, 12–15.

Wise, J. (2016). Hospitals and GPs are offered incentives to reduce antibiotic prescribing. *BMJ: British Medical Journal, 352.*

4

Nonpharmacological Aspects of Deprescribing

Deprescribing, like prescribing, can be regarded as a multifaceted intervention, and hence this chapter focuses on the major, anticipated nonpharmacological considerations. As touched upon in chapter 3, this may include real and imagined consequences for a patient, family and friends, treater, and systems (such as altered access to resources/entitlements). Lastly, this chapter will provide a method for anticipating, eliciting, and systematically addressing these concerns to prevent them from undermining the process of deprescribing.

Goal and Learning Objectives

After reading this chapter, the reader will be able to:

1. Outline the psycho-social-cultural factors and dynamics that underlie deprescribing
2. Identify patient roles, relationships, and resources that are need to be considered within a deprescribing plan
3. Describe strategies and a therapeutic stance for optimally managing these dynamics

The Psychological Meaning of Medications

The prescribing and ingestion of drugs is embedded in a matrix of cultural values and assumptions.

—Helman, 1981

We propose that deprescribing medications in the field of psychiatry requires the prescriber to consider not just the biological but also the psychological factors involved. Thus, a useful framework to apply is the psychodynamic meanings of medications as they relate to both the patient's inner and outer worlds. This outer world is constituted by significant others, friends and family, the prescriber and other mental health professionals, and even systems of care. A pill is not just a pill; the psychological meaning of taking the medication—or not taking the medication—must be incorporated into the deprescribing process. Failing to do so places the endeavor at risk of being undermined by unaddressed fears, concerns, needs, and associations. The symbolic meaning of medications, not only for the patient but also for the prescriber, the team, the family and broader society, should not be underestimated.

Rates of nonadherence to medications have been estimated at about 50–70% of patients with schizophrenia who do not take medication as prescribed (Bellack et al., 2009). Earlier research on what has been previously termed "noncompliance" to medication regimens provides some initial thoughts about the relationship of patient to medication. The issue of patients not taking medications as prescribed was first understood as a problem in the prescriber–patient relationship and/or problems in the patient's understanding of the illness (David, 1990). This has relevance to the "health belief" model, first suggested by Becker (1974), that suggested that patients are more likely to comply with a doctor's orders when they feel more at risk or susceptible to illness. However, on a more practical level, compliance is also found to increase when there are fewer perceived barriers such as cost or side effects.

The person-centered perspective on treatment considers patients to have a more active role in decision-making and is less focused on the "compliance" of the patient to the "orders" (Tondora, Miller, Slade, & Davidson, 2014). This perspective sees the patient as actively making decisions about what they feel is best for their body and their illness and focuses on an increase in self-determination and choice (Corrigan et al., 2012). The movement toward self-determination relates to an evolution in attitudes about the use of medication within the recovery movement. Within the recovery movement, medications are one of many possible tools in addressing mental illness, and their use relies on an authentic collaboration between prescriber and patient.

Perceived, intuited, or assumed biases on the part of the prescriber about medication may sway the patient's decision-making in either direction. A patient intent on pleasing the prescriber, or one who feels subjugated by, and fears retribution from, the prescriber, may superficially decide on a course of action with medication based on a wish to please. In other cases, *psychological reactance* (Brehm, 1966; Miron & Brehm, 2006), or a perceived threat to one's psychological autonomy in the face of requests or demands, may lead to a negating of any suggestions only out of a need to maintain a sense of coherence and personal will, rather than stemming from what is in the person's best interest.

Recent research into the impact of alliance and trauma further add to this picture. Tessier and colleagues (2017) found a correlation between higher levels of trauma in the psychiatric system and lower rates of adherence toward psychiatric medications. Adherence was increased by higher rates of alliance with the provider. This points to the importance of addressing traumatic experiences regarding the mental health system and could speak to the development of an "institutional transference" (Martin, 1989). With greater association of the medication to a perpetrator of trauma, if the medication in some way symbolizes the offending health care system, it would be intuitive to predict lower rates of adherence.

Medications act as symbols in cultural, economic, and psychic ways (Metzl & Riba, 2003). Antipsychotic medications, for instance, carry a cultural resonance related to controlling the behavior of those diagnosed with schizophrenia or other psychotic illnesses, based on assumptions regarding self-control and/or dangerousness. Some authors have suggested that medications themselves can be seen as entities that represent the sociocultural, economic, and technological trends of a given time period (Cohen, McCubbin, Collin, & Pérodeau, 2001). There is a "public protection" aspect to adherence with these medications, which may be reflected in discourse in the media. For example, an individual who presents as angry or uncontrolled may be referred to as "off their meds" in relaying a news story. This is an experience endorsed by patients who perceive medications as symbolizing a form of social control, as outlined in one study looking at those with schizophrenia (Rogers et al., 1998). From a psychoanalytic perspective, some writers have characterized medication as a third person in the therapeutic work, with patients' feelings about the therapist projected onto the medication (Tutter, 2006).

Even the act of taking a psychiatric medication for the first time is imbued with meaning and personal importance. Davidson (2001) describes his experience of first taking antidepressant medications as "a watershed event . . . [m]y hands shook as I opened the bottle for the first time". This intensity can be seen as representing a threshold crossing, from an identity as a 'well person' to that of someone with mental illness, with the medication acting as the vehicle for this transformation. Thus, stopping the medication can represent the return to health, if only symbolically. For some, stopping medication can feel like an important marker of recovery (Roe, Goldblatt, Baloush-Klienman, Swarbrick, & Davidson, 2008); this finding is important for its potential implications when returning to medications, as it may be challenging to restart a medication if it is seen as a "failure" or back-sliding from the patient's perspective. Taking a psychiatric medication can imply or confirm for some that they are truly ill; the medication is conflated with a diagnosis, and the message to one's self might be "if I'm taking medications, I must really be [crazy/sick/ill/insane]" (Swarbrick & Roe, 2011). Reversing this logic can be a motivator to stop medications, and understanding this motivation is crucial in providing accurate and specific support to a patient interested in deprescribing.

Mintz and colleagues have utilized the term *psychodynamic psychopharmacology* (Mintz, 2011; Mintz & Belnap, 2006) to describe the psychological aspects of the therapeutic relationship in reference to the use of medications. Mintz (2011) defines it as identifying the "central role of meaning and interpersonal factors in pharmacological treatment." In the description of resistance to taking medications, Mintz et al. say that it may be related to an unheard communication of the symptom and, with that, a reluctance to have it be silenced by the effects of medication. In extending this hypothesis to deprescribing, one can replace the symptom with the medication—if taking the medication symbolizes illness for a person, removing the medication may mean wellness or perceived wellness and a subsequent loss of care and concern by the prescriber, other caregivers, family, and friends.

These common dynamics identified in relation to medications and their meaning can provide insight into the reluctance to initiate deprescribing and help the prescriber to anticipate and understand unexpected or perplexing behavior. Box 4.1, excerpted from Mintz, Seery, and Cahill (2018), outlines some possible sources of harm from the meaning medications.

Patients may turn to medication as a way to avoid feeling or confronting difficult emotions. They may use medications as a way of pushing through

---

**Box 4.1 Examples of potential adverse effects
from medications that are mediated by meaning**

- Medications used to avoid responsibility or self-knowledge
- Medications used to avoid appropriate affect or healthy developmental steps
- Medications used to avoid acknowledgment of appropriate limitations
- Medications used to act out a traumatic scene
- Medications used to replace people
- Medications used to replace internal controls

Excerpted from Mintz et al. (2018).

---

and continuing on in situations that are untenable. For example, a person who becomes depressed and anxious in the context of an abusive romantic relationship may use antidepressants and anti-anxiety medications to avoid addressing the real context of a problematic relationship. Instead of approaching the situation head on, the medications are used as a way of addressing the distress without changing the situation. This form of resistance risks reducing potentially rich therapeutic encounters to simple transactions of symptom and dose.

Strategies to consider when approaching a situation that seems to be influenced by the countertherapeutic effects of medication are listed in Box 4.2 (Mintz et al., 2018).

Moving from a stance of dependence to autonomy, from patient to person, from consumer to independent actor—these shifts in self-perception and subsequent role changes are filled with meaning, ambivalence, and, at times, terror. While this often relates to fear of relapse or rehospitalization, these dynamics cut much deeper, potentially accessing historical roles and relationships such as being the *identified patient* in the family or social group. With this role unconsciously playing out, the deprescribing process may be unsuccessful due to unacknowledged feelings of betrayal on the part of the patient: "If I'm not sick, who will my mom have to take care of?" These dynamics that are often unconscious, require a significant trust in the relationship with the prescriber or other clinical provider to be comfortably explored in the process of deprescribing, and point to another reason why

---

Box 4.2 Deprescribing Strategies when Medications Have Meaning-Based Countertherapeutic Effects

---

- Develop an "overall diagnosis" that considers psychological aspects of treatment.
- Focus on the therapeutic alliance.
- Ameliorate harm by addressing pathogenic meanings.
- Consider countertransferential contributions to the impulse to deprescribe.
- Approach deprescribing as an interpersonal process.
- Attend to the treatment context.
- Deprescribe in a planful way that maximizes patient learning and authority.
- Consider that it is better to give no treatment than bad treatment.

Excerpted from Mintz et al. (2018).

---

the process of deprescribing may need to take place over a significant length of time, with potentially several "false starts" and reconsiderations as these dynamics begin to emerge more clearly.

How to Elicit Significant Psychological Factors when Deprescribing

Eliciting concerns about deprescribing needs to be done carefully and with the consideration that patients may not be consciously aware of the meanings they ascribe to the use of medication, and, even if they are aware, it might be less acceptable to acknowledge these meanings. Approaching these questions in a gentle and nonjudgmental way, and within one's own psychotherapeutic frame and proficiencies, is of essential importance. A focus on the relationship and addressing any ruptures in the alliance as the conversation moves forward provides a good foundation.

As much as possible, the idea that the patient is using the medication as a way of avoiding strong emotion must be approached in a strengths-based way; for example, by framing this use of medications as an adaptation to a difficult circumstance when no other tools were available to the person. A nonshaming approach, contextualizing the history and social dynamics of a person's life, can place the use of medications in a temporal context that serves to explain their previous usefulness and potential loss of such function in the present day. This is similar to any coping skill or defense once utilized successfully and that now, having outgrown or outlived its use, needs to be shifted and exchanged for something else.

The use of medications may be a way of reinforcing "patienthood" (Mintz, 2011). The idea of medications being a message that a person is ill and perhaps not responsible for their actions or behaviors can be a barrier to deprescribing, depending on the dynamic functioning of this stance in a person's life. There may be certain fears associated with being something other than a "patient," - fears that have been reinforced over the years due to the negative consequences of previous deprescribing trials or other negative experiences of trying to venture out beyond patienthood. Particularly vulnerable are those who have been institution-alized or part of the mental health system for a long period of time. Even when the prescriber sees the medications as potentially more harmful than beneficial and may be interested in starting a conversation about the reduction of one of these medications, the patient may be opposed for reasons not initially clear; this is an important prompt for further exploration.

Attending to the alliance and therapeutic relationship is a crucial ele-ment in understanding meaning and laying foundations for moving for-ward with any deprescribing effort. The alliance is considered the best predictor of outcomes in therapeutic efforts (Martin, Garske, & Davis, 2000). Adherence studies have identified the relationship with the pro-vider as a positive predictor of adherence to prescribed regimens (Day et al., 2005) and perceived coercion as a negative predictor of adher-ence. Focusing on identifying if any dynamics (perhaps related to power differentials, early parental relationships or past history in the present re-lationship) are playing out around the medication is important to consider in the process. In addition, it is important to acknowledge that there may be multiple and potentially contradictory dynamics playing out, without becoming wed to a single understanding, as relationships are changing and context-dependent.

The Sociocultural Significance of Medications

As discussed briefly in Chapter 3 around identity disruption as a barrier to deprescribing, a medication regimen may be perceived by patients or social supports as a "badge of illness" or indeed as "membership" in social groups from which patients derive significant support and enjoyment. For example, a patient with schizophrenia who attends weekly clozapine medication group as one of their most significant social interactions, and who deeply values the camaraderie she experiences there, may be reluctant to give up that particular medication due to the medication-specific social benefits. Similarly, a patient who has grown fond of their visiting nurse, who they have seen daily for medication administration for the past several years, may do poorly in a deprescribing effort solely due to a nonpharmacological effect—the significant loss of social contact through nursing visits. Efforts may be made to identify the potential for support and to grieve any losses. Alternative supports may be found, or advocacy for exceptions/policy change in local care systems, may be appropriate. Systems and payers of care might consider reframing group membership and eligibility for services to better acknowledge those in recovery without medications.

The simple ritual of periodically refilling and taking a medication may be significant to some patients. Social interactions, prompts for general wellness maintenance (e.g., personal hygiene or flu vaccination), and earlier detection of burgeoning medical illness may be collateral benefits of a monthly visit to the pharmacy. These effects may be difficult to detect in advance; strategies might include a detailed step-by-step walk-through of a patient's everyday activities or asking them to imagine impacts on their routine if no longer taking the medication.

Cultural differences in attitudes and practices related to medications have been reported but should not be assumed solely based on group membership. An exploration (involving collaterals) may illuminate relevant factors in an individual culture or subculture biasing toward or against a deprescribing. Medication side effects may be experienced as meaningful or a marker of efficacy. Depending on cultural factors, a patient revealing multiple prescriptions may elicit increased concern and caregiving as readily as being perceived as inferior and ostracizing. The relationship between the allopathic prescription and alternative, natural, or traditional remedies should also be considered. The response in a patient's cultural environment to a deprescribing might include the reciprocal refocusing on such remedies for better or for worse.

On a systems level, risks of losing entitlements or resources, either real or perceived, may undermine deprescribing. These risks may be mitigated with time as deprescribing becomes more prominent as a treatment intervention. Until then, however, it is easy to imagine that a reviewer of a disability application might more readily associate an applicant with an extensive list of high-dose medications with greater severity of illness (and therefore disability) than an individual on a single minimum effective dose medication who preferentially leverages psychosocial treatments. If a valid presumption, this will likely be amenable to education and advocacy.

Conclusion

Considering the psychological meaning and sociocultural significance of medications is an important part of prescribing but can be especially salient when deprescribing. Previously incomprehensible behaviors may become clearer and more understandable when seen through the lens of psychic meaning and the polarities of care versus neglect, health versus illness (and other identity markers or role designations). Group memberships, entitlements, and access to resources may be challenged.

Nonpharmacological concerns, once elicited and examined, may contribute positively to the process of deprescribing and may have the unintended positive result of identifying previously unaddressed dynamics and opportunities for further social recovery for the patient. Approaching these questions with care, concern, and attention to the alliance will best support this exploration of often difficult dynamics. If a prescriber identifies limitations due to time or training/supervision, it would be appropriate to engage a psychotherapist to collaborate in support of deprescribing.

Case Examples

Case Example 1

Josh is a 55-year-old, single, unemployed man taking haloperidol decanoate injections, divalproex, gabapentin, and benztropine. He has a history of drinking heavily and using crack cocaine in his 30s, following which he was admitted to a long-term state hospital for more than 2 years. He has no complaints except for a generalized tremor that subsided after discontinuing divalproex. Following this, the gabapentin and benztropine were also slowly discontinued as the indication for their use was unclear. He seemed slightly more talkative but not disruptive. Several months into the deprescribing trial, he lost his temper with his case manager, after realizing that she had been skimming money from his slim disability income, and yelled at a neighbor because of his smoking crack in Josh's apartment building. These outbursts caused Josh to be hospitalized, following which the divalproex was restarted. On return to the outpatient clinic, he declined the divalproex and had the support of his psychiatrist and therapist to stay off the medication. In subsequent sessions with his therapist, he revealed for the first time, an instance where he was sexually abused by the family pastor. This revelation, when shared with his brother, led to an altercation between the two of them and, eventually, to another hospitalization. This time, however, Josh did not return to the outpatient clinic after discharge and was not in contact for more than 4 months. When he did return, Josh said that he had spent the summer in a larger, nearby city and was feeling quite well. He had, however, lost his subsidized apartment, lost any contact with his brother, and lost contact with a visiting nurse whom he cherished. He admitted to having drank alcohol but had not used crack. He had been to the emergency room of a hospital in the nearby city and had been given a large dose of haloperidol decanoate on one occasion. Josh also added that he was afraid he would lose his disability income if he was not prescribed enough medication. He also wondered if divalproex was actually "good for him," and he was placed on haloperidol and divalproex again. Interestingly, the level of divalproex was found to be very low every time it was subsequently measured. Over the next year, Josh asked for the divalproex to be stopped and asked for a higher dose of haloperidol.

During this period, he used crack cocaine a few times, was hospitalized twice, but was more engaged in both group and individual therapy. He referred to the sexual trauma a few times and seemed to be on his way to eventually processing it.

This example illustrates the numerous identity and social issues that may arise during deprescribing (indeed as they can during prescribing). These issues, such as being taken advantage of by his case manager, and the revelation of the sexual trauma, were not immediately obvious in the manner in which this individual's life progressed, but seemed to underlie some of his actions and those of the people surrounding him.

The first issue that arises is his relatively desirable response to the deprescribing of the divalproex, gabapentin and benztropine. He seemed more cheerful and happier. For an individual who has been "awarded" a lifetime diagnosis of schizophrenia and thus been "sentenced" to a lifetime of medication, what did it mean that, to Josh, he was *well*, and even better, without many of his medications? Along with feeling less sedated overall, he seemed to have reconnected with an identity that had presumably diffused at the start of his psychosis, and been reconstituted as that of a "schizophrenic" and as a "consumer" of medications. This illness identity seemed to diffuse again with the suggestion that he may not need that many medications after all.

The second phenomenon that emerged was a realization of a sense of agency and that Josh recognized himself as a potential source of action and as the recipient of the consequences of his actions. This manifested itself in Josh addressing his difficulties with his case manager and his neighbor, and subsequently, in one interpretation, being punished (with a hospitalization) for exercising his right to defend and protect himself. While his reactions may have not been the most socially acceptable, the reaction (of being hospitalized) to his increase in agency may point to lingering stigma and discrimination within the mental health system, where healthy agency among someone diagnosed with schizophrenia can be construed as symptomatic and requiring treatment. The uncovering of the sexual trauma and the ensuing shame and anger led to altercations with his brother and another visit to the hospital. The hospitalization could be considered an illustration of the mobilization of social forces, including his brother, his housing agency (that placed the emergency call), and mental health professionals to "keep Josh in his place."

In this example, divalproex, in Josh's mind, had become the ticket to retaining his disability income and perhaps even retaining a relationship with his brother. He, however, disliked feeling affectless and sleepy and did not wish to take it. This conflict about divalproex appeared in his requesting a prescription but not really consuming the medication. The concern over losing his benefits and his brother was heightened by the advice from friends and his brother's refusal to see him "without your meds."

Similar to shifts in family dynamics when an identified "alcoholic" first enters recovery, Josh's family role, as passive 'schizophrenic', was shifting with his reduction in medication, causing ripple effects in other relationships including that with the mental health system. The question around the flexibility of the mental health system itself to be able to support a patient as their role and identity shifts also emerges in this scenario. This is something to be sensitive to within the context of deprescribing; that, despite the prescriber's best efforts to flexibly and individually conduct a deprescribing trial, larger systems (e.g. familial or social) may push back against these changes if only as an attempt to reestablish equilibrium.

Case Example 2

Gina is a 57-year-old heterosexual woman, divorced, unemployed, living alone in an apartment. She was taking risperidone, benztropine, occasional diphenhydramine, and a small dose of lithium that could be considered subtherapeutic based on blood level. Gina was assigned to a prescriber who had newly joined the practice following the retirement of a colleague. She appreciated the new prescriber, who she felt was not very focused on medication but who wanted to talk to her. On one visit, the prescriber mentioned to her that she didn't need the lithium and was discontinuing it. After 2 weeks, Gina informed the office that she was having anxiety and that she needed to take lithium. The prescriber offered to increase the dose of diphenhydramine and pointed out several ways in which the lithium was not suitable for her anymore, but she would not agree and continued to be determined to restart the lithium. She had mentioned several times to the new prescriber that Dr. James had prescribed the lithium more than 20 years ago and that her ex-husband frequently taunted her saying "are you off your lithium again?" whenever she lost her temper or laughed loudly.

Gina's attachment to the lithium and refusal to stop taking it, despite a low possibility of therapeutic benefit (or withdrawal symptoms) indicated that there were unidentified factors at play that were mediating her anxiety. Although she did not make the connection between the two, her anxiety over the discontinuation of lithium could be related to the departure of Dr. James who had treated her for more than 20 years. Discontinuing the lithium, to her, was like severing her last connection with a prescriber whom she trusted and valued. Further, her ex-husband's repeated taunts led to a conclusion about herself that "unmedicated Gina" was intolerable and deserved to be mocked or punished. She had internalized the idea that the only way to be acceptable to society was to take lithium. With this hypothesized link between the medication and the relationship with her previous doctor, addressing the grief over losing Dr. James and what it means to now "go against" his recommendations may free Gina to try reducing the lithium. The treatment team may also assist Gina in seeing herself as a person of worth even without the lithium, supporting her in beginning to undo the damage caused by her husband's comments. Both these issues if addressed before the medication itself is changed will likely promote a more successful trial off the lithium. Furthermore, the unilateral decision to stop the lithium made by her new prescriber may have triggered psychological reactance; the sense that her autonomy was compromised may have foreclosed the deprescribing option for Gina. Including Gina in the initial decision-making and eliciting these concerns about loyalty to her previous doctor and the characterization of her by her ex-husband may have better allowed Gina and her prescriber to better understand and therefore address these concerns and dynamics on the front end.

Self-Assessment

1. Which of the following dynamics may become activated by a suggestion of deprescribing?
   a. Relinquishing the role of the "identified patient"
   b. Fears around a greater sense of agency
   c. Fear of repercussions on relationships with significant others
   d. All of the above

Correct answer: **d.** All of the above.

2. Which of the following may compel a patient to decline changes in medication?
   a. Fear of relapse/rehospitalization/incarceration
   b. Ritualization of the process of obtaining and consuming medication and building a social circle around it
   c. Fear of not looking ill enough on an application for benefits
   d. All of the above
   e. None of the above

Correct answer: **d.** All of the above.

3. Which of the following may be a social implication of deprescribing?
   a. Threat of divorce from spouse
   b. Family cutting off communication
   c. Kidney problems
   d. Only a
   e. A and b

Correct answer: **e.** A and b.

References

Becker, M. H. (1974). The health belief model and sick role behavior. *Health Education Monographs*, 2(4), 409–419.

Bellack, A. S., Bowden, C. L., Bowie, C. R., Byerly, M. J., Carpenter, W. T., Copeland, L. A., . . . Diaz, E. (2009). The expert consensus guideline series: Adherence problems in patients with serious and persistent mental illness. *Journal of Clinical Psychiatry*, 70(Suppl. 4), 1–48.

Brehm, J. W. (1966). *A Theory of Psychological Reactance*. Oxford: Academic Press.

Cohen, D., McCubbin, M., Collin, J., & Pérodeau, G. (2001). Medications as social phenomena. *Health*, *5*(4), 441–469. doi:10.1177/136345930100 500403.

Corrigan, P. W., Angell, B., Davidson, L., Marcus, S. C., Salzer, M. S., Kottsieper, P., . . . Stanhope, V. (2012). From adherence to self-determination: Evolution of a treatment paradigm for people with serious mental illnesses. *Psychiatric Services*, *63*(2), 169–173. doi:10.1176/appi.ps.201100065.

David, A. S. (1990). Insight and psychosis. *The British Journal of Psychiatry*, *156*(6), 798–808.

Davidson, L. (2001). Personal accounts: Us and them. *Psychiatric Services*, *52*(12), 1579–1580. doi:10.1176/appi.ps.52.12.1579.

Day, J. C., Bentall, R. P., Roberts, C., Randall, F., Rogers, A., Cattell, D., . . . Power, C. (2005). Attitudes toward antipsychotic medication: The impact of clinical variables and relationships with health professionals. *Archives of General Psychiatry*, *62*(7), 717–724. doi:10.1001/archpsyc.62.7.717.

Helman, C. G. (1981). 'Tonic', 'fuel' and 'food': Social and symbolic aspects of the long-term use of psychotropic drugs. *Social Science & Medicine. Part B: Medical Anthropology*, *15*(4), 521–533. doi:https://doi.org/10.1016/ 0160-7987(81)90026-0.

Martin, D. J., Garske, J. P., & Davis, M. K. (2000). Relation of the therapeutic alliance with outcome and other variables: A meta-analytic review. *Journal of Consulting and Clinical Psychology*, *68*(3), 438–450.

Martin, H. P. (1989). Types of institutional transference. *Bulletin of the Menninger Clinic*, *53*(1), 58–62.

Metzl, J. M., & Riba, M. (2003). Understanding the symbolic value of medications: A brief review. *Primary Psychiatry*, *10*(7), 45–64.

Mintz, D. (2011). Psychodynamic psychopharmacology: Addressing the underlying causes of treatment resistance. *Psychiatric Times*, *28*(9), 22.

Mintz, D., & Belnap, B. (2006). A view from Riggs: Treatment resistance and patient authority—III. What is psychodynamic psychopharmacology? An approach to pharmacologic treatment resistance. *Journal of the American Academy of Psychoanalysis and Dynamic Psychiatry*, *34*(4), 581–601. doi:10.1521/jaap.2006.34.4.581.

Mintz, D., Seery, E., & Cahill, J. (2018). Deprescribing: A psychodynamically-informed, patient-centered perspective. *Current Psychiatry Reviews*, *14*(1), 19–25. doi:10.2174/1573400514666180524095024.

Miron, A. M., & Brehm, J. W. (2006). Reactance theory—40 years later. *Zeitschrift für Sozialpsychologie, 37*(1), 9–18. doi:10.1024/0044–3514.37.1.9.

Roe, D., Goldblatt, H., Baloush-Klienman, V., Swarbrick, M., & Davidson, L. (2008). Why and how people decide to stop taking prescribed psychiatric medication: Exploring the subjective process of choice. *Psychiatric Rehabilitation Journal, 33*(1), 38–46.

Rogers, A., Day, J. C., Williams, B., Randall, F., Wood, P., Healy, D., & Bentall, R. P. (1998). The meaning and management of neuroleptic medication: A study of patients with a diagnosis of schizophrenia. *Social Science & Medicine, 47*(9), 1313–1323. doi:https://doi.org/10.1016/S0277-9536(98)00209-3.

Swarbrick, M., & Roe, D. (2011). Experiences and motives relative to psychiatric medication choice. *Psychiatric Rehabilitation Journal, 35*(1), 45.

Tessier, A., Boyer, L., Husky, M., Baylé, F., Llorca, P.-M., & Misdrahi, D. (2017). Medication adherence in schizophrenia: The role of insight, therapeutic alliance and perceived trauma associated with psychiatric care. *Psychiatry Research, 257*, 315–321. doi:https://doi.org/10.1016/j.psychres.2017.07.063.

Tondora, J., Miller, R., Slade, M., & Davidson, L. (2014). *Partnering for Recovery in Mental Health: A Practical Guide to Person-Centered Planning.* New York: John Wiley & Sons.

Tutter, A. (2006). Medication as object. *Journal of the American Psychoanalytic Association, 54*(3), 781–804.

PART 2
THE INTERVENTION
OF DEPRESCRIBING

5

Wellness Approaches I

Self-Determined Strategies

It is important for deprescribing not to be experienced as a withdrawal of treatment per se and certainly not withdrawal of care or concern on the part of the treater. A key element of this is acknowledging and bolstering of existing strategies or the introduction and development of new strategies for maintaining wellness. These can come solely from the patient and their social supports or in collaboration with treaters. This chapter addresses wellness supports that may be suggested by the prescriber but are essentially put in place by the patient to *support* a deprescribing process. These strategies are not being proposed here as *replacements* for the indicated pharmacotherapy, or as standalone treatments for any given diagnosis as a multi-dimensional approach remains key. In the same way we neither encourage, nor recommend, flight to these non-pharmaceutical strategies to justify a reactive abandonment of pharmacotherapy.

This chapter discusses the management of one of the major concerns about deprescribing raised by patients, prescribers, and family members alike—namely, *relapse*, or a return of symptoms that can impact a person's quality of life. While a return of symptoms may or may not necessitate a return to medication, other alternative strategies put in place might prevent or best manage an increase in distress. The focus is on a wellness approach and personal wellness strategies. These include two well-recognized self-management strategies: the development of a Wellness Recovery Action Plan (WRAP), which is an evidence-based practice that includes a person's own identified "toolbox" of daily self-management strategies, and the use of "personal medicine," which is a group of strategies that are self-initiated, nonpharmaceutical self-care activities. Even if the prescriber is not participating directly in these activities, we argue that it is beneficial to show interest and awareness of these strategies in order to support the alliance and avoid reinforcing mind-body splits which may occur for the patient, projected between members of the treatment team. Potentially detrimental, these mind body splits could hinder the integration of care/'work' the patient undertakes alone, with their therapist or with their prescriber, for example. Assuming some readers will be less familiar with this area, we include in this chapter a targeted review of the literature.

Goal and Learning Objectives

After reading this chapter, the reader will be able to:

1. Name at least five personal supports to consider for someone interested in deprescribing
2. Identify two benefits of implementing self-management strategies
3. Describe WRAP and personal medicine as they can be used to support deprescribing.

Adopting a Wellness Approach

Using Swarbrick's (2006) definition of a *wellness approach*, the deprescribing provider will benefit from taking a holistic, multidimensional look at the patient, with the focus being on areas of strength, health, and vitality in order to maximize the effectiveness of deprescribing and to collaborate with them from a recovery-oriented perspective. Moving away from a strict focus on symptoms and instead adopting a stance of what best supports a person's quality of life and pursuit of valued life goals can change the focus on symptom and illness to a more pragmatic "what works" stance. Increasingly in health care, and especially in psychiatry, there is growing evidence and support for "self-management" strategies to support an individual's own role in staying well.

This focus on progress in important areas of a person's life includes identifying things such as purpose, friends and family, work, hobbies, and other valued actions (including giving back to the community and contributing to family and organizations). In fact, a recent study looking at patients' stated reasons for seeking medications showed that 51% identified "social relationships" as the goal for their medication use, and they saw medications overall as a support toward pursuing valued life goals.

Interestingly, in this sample of patients, 31% also identified reducing or stopping medications as their goal in meeting with their prescriber (Deegan et al., 2017). Increasing this focus on wellness is an important element in starting a deprescribing trial.

It is especially important to keep a wellness approach in mind when thinking about deprescribing because, within this process, the fear of "relapse" or return of psychiatric symptoms can be a terrifying notion for all involved (including the patient and their family as well as the care team and the prescriber), as discussed in Chapter 3 when considering barriers to deprescribing. Through various adjunctive supports and approaches, including *preplanning and crisis planning, peer support, social support,* and other forms of "*personal medicine,*" adjunctive avenues can decrease the need for pharmacological intervention and support the process of deprescribing. What follows briefly outlines each of these categories and how each might be integrated on an individual basis for persons interested in deprescribing.

Planning Ahead for Relapse

Identifying the early warning signs of relapse is particularly important when initiating a deprescribing process. Even if we are successful at redefining relapse, expanding the notion of health, approaching a person in a recovery-oriented manner, and destigmatizing hospitalization; these experiences are still potentially best avoided not only because of the distress they cause, but also for the potentially major life disruption and loss of time and income for the person. Identifying early warning signs or predictors of relapse is not clear-cut from a research perspective, but scales such as the Early Symptom Scale can reliably predict a relapse and facilitate effective secondary prevention (Birchwood et al., 1989).

One of the key practices, therefore, in deprescribing, is creating a plan in advance that describes how the prescriber, patient, and other identified members of the team will respond when there is an increase in distress or symptoms or a significant change in functioning. This team may include family members; friends; the pastor, imam, or other spiritual leader; the visiting nurse; a peer support staff; or someone else named by the person as vital to their path to recovery and wellness. A plan may be formalized, written, and contain many detailed specifics and steps. Alternatively, the plan may be more straightforward, with only a few key actions to be taken. Legal and quasi-legal documents, including advance directives and documents of treatment preference, can set out in advance a *roadmap* to guide the person and their team when symptoms increase and/or health and function declines.

Psychiatric Advance Directive

There are a number of existing treatment planning tools to help patients articulate preferences during more difficult times (i.e., when preoccupied by symptoms or unable to competently make or indicate choices). At one end of the spectrum is a *psychiatric advance directive* (PAD), which is a potentially legally enforceable documentation of a person's preferences, wishes, and choices (O'Connell, 2015). This is particularly important for those people who, when more symptomatic, may become unable to express their wishes or may behave in ways that would be distressing to them in other nonsymptomatic states. In order to construct such a document, a person must do so at a time when they are considered capable of making decisions and articulating preferences for treatment.

For example, a 32-year-old woman with bipolar disorder, when depressed, also becomes psychotic and virtually mute. She communicates only in metaphor and is unable to express her needs. When well, she clearly knows her preferences for which hospital, medication, and course of treatment she finds acceptable or unacceptable. For example, she consents in her PAD to electroconvulsive therapy only in the instance that (1) alternative indicated approaches have been unsuccessful and (2) she is actively suicidal with imminent risk. These specific wishes are clearly articulated and include great detail, such as stating that she is willing to take trifluoperazine but not haloperidol for psychotic symptoms due to prior experience with those medications (a history of side effects).

The detailing of these preferences is important for several reasons. In relation to deprescribing, patients may leave an inpatient admission prescribed multiple new medications with which they do not have buy-in and that future prescribers are reluctant to change. A detailed plan can include which medications are preferred and have been useful in the past, as well as those which are not preferred due to either side effects or being ineffective in the past. This may prevent unnecessary medications from being initiated at times of crisis and thereby circumvent the need for a deprescribing intervention down the line.

In addition, creating such a plan can help the person with mental illness to feel more in control and empowered around the experience of hospitalization or the experience of an increase in symptoms. PADs have been shown to reduce the number of coercive interventions in a crisis, which can in turn lead to less trauma and greater trust and empowerment in the person with mental illness (Swanson et al., 2008).

Other planning tools to support a person in outlining preferences are readily available as templates and guidelines to help a person catch, as early as possible, a serious symptom recurrence. One example is a crisis planning tool from the State of Maine Department of Mental Health (State of Maine Substance Abuse and Mental Health Services, 2016) and a tool used in behavioral health services in Oregon (Oregon Behavioral Health Network, 2016). As a more progressive and sociocultural focused example, the Icarus Project has developed what they term "Mad Maps," which include identifying sources of oppression and creating a self-directed wellness and empowerment tool (DeBrul & The Icarus Project, 2015). In the United Kingdom, the National Institute for Health and Care Excellence outlines what it has identified as the key elements of any crisis plan, as listed in Box 5.1.

These guidelines can serve as an outline for information and decisions that are helpful to make in advance of any deprescribing intervention.

Wellness Recovery Action Plan

Another evidence-based intervention related to planning ahead is that of the Wellness Recovery Action Plan (WRAP; Copeland, 1997), a peer-led or individually implemented intervention which grew out of Copeland's research with people who mobilized wellness strategies to maintain health either on or off medications. Copeland interviewed a number of people to categorize helpful approaches to living with mental illnesses; from this work, she created a now world-recognized curriculum to support people in identifying their own key strategies for staying well. Based on the lived experience of people with mental illness, the WRAP curriculum guides one through identifying what one needs to do on a daily basis to stay well (the wellness toolbox), including basic self-care approaches like, "get 8 hours

---

Box 5.1 Guidelines for Advance Plan Development

1. Possible early warning signs of a crisis and coping strategies
2. Support available to help prevent hospitalization
3. Where the person would like to be admitted in the event of hospitalization
4. The practical needs of the service user if they are admitted to hospital (e.g., childcare or the care of other dependents, including pets)
5. Details of advance statements and advance decisions
6. Whether and the degree to which families or carers are involved
7. Information about 24-hour access to services
8. Named contacts

From National Institute of Health and Care Excellence (2016).

---

of sleep," "eat breakfast," and "talk to a friend." These simple but powerful strategies support people in taking control of their well-being and having lists and ideas on hand to refer to when things are not going well. Along with the wellness toolbox, WRAP assists in identifying "early warning signs"; those small but important behavioral markers that a relapse may be more likely. These signs are highly individualized; for example, one person identified that when she stopped looking to cross the street, she knew that she needed to do more to take care of herself. Identifying these signs can be a collaborative process with the prescriber and the patient, particularly around deprescribing interventions.

Identifying early warning signs can also be done with peer support or a friend or family member. Having a sense of what to look for, and what others should look for, can again help empower the person, allow them to feel more in control of their symptoms, and have the sense of having a "safety net." WRAP also includes a crisis planning tool, similar but potentially more detailed than a PAD. The crisis planning tool guides the identification of specific preferences around medications, hospitals, and any other instructions designed to support a person in crisis when they may not be able to articulate their own wishes. WRAP is generally conducted in groups led by peer support staff but can be done individually and online. The WRAP plan should never be required to be shared with the prescriber nor other clinical team members as this goes against the ethos of a self-determined and -owned wellness plan (Copeland, 1997). But encouraging the person to share aspects of the plan, if not the whole plan, can be beneficial because it contains rich clinical material. The early warning signs can be crucial in identifying and potentially averting relapse during the deprescribing process. The prescriber may be able to discern some of these from previous episodes and from discussion with family and other clinical providers, as well as (and most importantly) through discussion with the patient herself.

Research evidence regarding WRAP shows that it produces significant symptom reduction, increases hope and recovery, and has a positive impact on perceived physical health. Counter-intuitively however, empowerment scores appeared to decrease in this study (Cook et al., 2009). A randomized clinical trial found similar results, including an overall reduction in symptom severity, an increase in hope, and an increase in quality of life (Cook et al., 2011). WRAP is based on principles of empowerment theory and self-efficacy (Bandura, 1977).

Personal Medicine

Another useful concept to introduce in the context of deprescribing, and particularly for those patients who may be attached to the idea of medication, is "personal medicine," a term coined by Deegan (2005). As a psychologist who identifies as having schizophrenia, she has worked to develop tools to support greater empowerment of people around their treatment. Personal medicine comprises strategies that are "self-initiated, non-pharmaceutical self-care activities that served to decrease symptoms, avoid undesirable outcomes such as hospitalization, and improve mood, thoughts, behaviors, and overall sense of wellbeing" (Deegan, 2005, p. 3). Identifying these strategies and supporting people in practicing them can be a role played in part by the prescriber as well as by other members of the clinical team and/or family and friends. Gaining a sense of control or increasing self-efficacy can be an empowering experience, supporting increased self-esteem and confidence in the process of managing illness. For the prescriber in their collaboration with the patient, support around identifying these strategies is essential to providing additional personal resources and strategies to manage the potential psychological stress arising from reduction of medication (i.e., fear of relapse) and to manage a possible increase in symptoms resulting from the reduced use of medication.

In deprescribing, advance directives and other planning tools can be helpful not only in providing concrete suggestions for action and specific preferences for treatment that are in line with the person's wishes, but the planning itself also provides somewhat of a psychological safety net for the person: having these things spelled out and having the document (whether it be a PAD, a crisis plan, or a WRAP) in the hands of natural supports (such as family, friends, the prescriber) can act as reassurance that things are in place in case something does happen. The process of creating an advanced plan can also be empowering for the person and stimulate previously undiscussed topics with friends and family about what the person would prefer to have happen in the case of a reemergence of symptoms. For many people with serious mental illness, as with anyone, having something in place to take care of children, pets, or plants that depend on them is essential. Patients may refuse inpatient care because, for example, there may be no one in place to take care of their beloved dog or to water their prized plants. With a plan in place, a person can feel freer to address their own needs and go into the hospital if needed without the added stress of worrying about their children, companion animals, or plants.

An important critique about the use of WRAP and other self-management strategies is the commentary by Scott (2005), which states that these strategies continue to promote a deficit-based identity despite their potential usefulness. This is important to consider when promoting something such as WRAP, because a patient may need to process the idea that being able to control the illness does not also imply that they are somehow responsible for causing it. Self-management approaches can also inadvertently have the unintended consequence of leading to a kind of hypervigilance around any change in mood or thoughts. The fear of relapse and the promotion of self-monitoring for any signs of this can lead to a foreclosure of natural mood variation and a limiting of experience in order to maintain a kind of ill-conceived sense of "stability." Instead, the goal of recovery-oriented approaches such as WRAP and other self-management strategies is to promote a sense of hope, empowerment, and reduction of distress in order to allow the pursuit of valued life goals and to increase meaning and purpose in life.

Meaning and Purpose

Meaning and purpose in life is considered a valued aspect of recovery-oriented care and is a well-researched aspect of well-being. The positive psychology field lends support to the importance of having meaning and purpose in one's life. One early study confirmed this association between purpose in life and psychological well-being (Zika & Chamberlain, 1992). The literature on stress resilience also supports finding and pursuing meaningful life activities as a way to moderate and manage stress.

Exercise

The literature supporting exercise as an intervention, particularly in affective disorders, continues to grow (see Greer & Trivedi, 2009). Despite the caveat that rigorous studies of more controlled samples of subjects are warranted, current evidence supports exercise as a treatment for mild to moderate depression, as confirmed in several meta-analyses (see Cooney, Dwan, & Mead, 2014; Knapen, Vancampfort, Moriën, & Marchal, 2015).

There is also a growing literature supporting the adjunctive use of exercise in schizophrenia. Exercise may contribute to a reduction in symptoms of schizophrenia (Scheewe et al., 2013). Another review of three randomized controlled trials showed significant reduction of negative symptoms, but not positive symptoms, when looking at the effects of exercise (Gorczynski & Faulkner, 2010). A meta-analysis found exercise benefits for people with schizophrenia in reducing symptoms and improving functioning and neurocognition with a dose of at least 90 minutes of moderate exercise a week (Firth, Cotter, Elliott, French, & Yung, 2015). A more recent meta-analysis found that exercise reduced symptoms and improved quality of life in those with depression and schizophrenia (Dauwan, Begemann, Heringa, & Sommer, 2016). Evidence for exercise continues to grow and can be recommended as a possible addition to a deprescribing endeavor.

Family Support

Strong evidence for the contributions of family therapy to the multi-dimensional care of schizophrenia comes in particular from McFarlane's studies on multifamily groups (McFarlane, 2002). There is some evidence for relapse prevention particularly with single family therapy (Pilling et al., 2002).

One long-validated predictor of relapse in people with bipolar disorder and schizophrenia has been the concept of *expressed emotion* (EE) in families. EE is defined as emotional overinvolvement and critical communication from family members or significant others. A meta-analysis identified levels of EE as a robust predictor of relapse in schizophrenia, mood disorders, and eating disorders (Butzlaff & Hooley, 1998). A recent 20-year follow-up study found higher rates of relapse and hospitalizations as well as positive symptoms in those people with families high in EE (Cechnicki, Bielańska, Hanuszkiewicz, & Daren, 2013). Family interventions, therefore, are strongly recommended to support family education around mental illness and particularly to assist families in reducing levels of EE (Pharoah, Mari, Rathbone, & Wong, 2010). This is particularly relevant in deprescribing and may be an adjunctive component to add to the treatment and supports needed to help prevent increases in symptoms that may be exacerbated by family dynamics. Family therapy is especially a consideration for those patients living at home, younger adults, and those with family members serving as legal conservators.

In a review of family-based strategies in preventing relapse for people with mental illness, Falloon (2003) analyzed 50 studies from 1980 onward. Studies were diverse in their interventions, but findings indicated that in those studies combining medication management and case management with or without family stress management, those with stress management showed clinical improvement in 14 out of 18 studies. One meta-analysis found that critical comments by caregivers (negative expressed emotions) increased the likelihood of relapse by 2.2 times in first-episode psychosis (Alvarez-Jimenez et al., 2012).

In a unique book, Mackler and Morrissey (2010) detail recommendations for "dealing with your family after you've been diagnosed with a psychiatric disorder." This brief, practical book covers family roles, boundaries, family conflict, and other areas vital to address for the person in recovery, along with personal accounts of family experiences. Each chapter also includes questions for self-reflection that encourage a critical and thoughtful approach to self and others. This is one example of using what is sometimes termed *bibliotherapy*: using books as tools in managing mental health. Personal accounts (cf. Jamison, 1995; Saks, 2007) are also useful for some, serving as inspiration and role modelling around living with a mental illness.

Novel and Progressive Approaches

Emerging paradigms such as the Hearing Voices movement (see Corstens, Longden, McCarthy-Jones, Waddingham, & Thomas, 2014; Styron, Utter, & Davidson, 2017) and other alternative views of psychopathology as "extreme states" would challenge the designation of an increase in symptoms as a relapse per se. In this paradigm, an increase in voices or other "symptoms" (in quotes to emphasize the paradigm's ambivalence if not rejection of this term) might be seen as important data about life circumstances (unaddressed anger, problematic relationships) that need to be addressed or changed, in contrast to being seen as a flare up of an underlying autonomous disease process. In qualitative research, people who hear voices identified the personal context and understanding of such (the personal meaning and understanding of voice hearing) to be most beneficial to coping with and adapting to hearing voices (Corstens et al., 2014).

Alternative views of psychopathology can be accessed in mutual support groups. In particular, the Alternatives to Suicide and the Hearing Voices Network groups are two to highlight as innovative and potentially not as well-known to providers. Hearing Voices groups do not necessarily characterize these experiences as symptoms to reduce or eliminate. Instead, the groups and the philosophy of the approach, conceptualize voices as part of the continuum of human experience and as experiences with meaning to potentially be understood by the voice hearer. One facet is that many, if not most, people who hear voices have experiences of trauma and that understanding the voices can be helpful in reducing distress (Dillon & Longden, 2013). Groups provide a sense of containment, new relationships, and greater understanding of voice-hearing (Payne, Allen, & Lavender, 2017). Learning from others' personal stories and experiences is an essential part of the approach, and some of these stories were put together in a volume *Living with Voices: 50 Stories of Recovery* (Romme, Escher, Dillon, Corstens, & Morris, 2009) that provides a diverse range of accounts. Research on Hearing Voices groups is in preliminary stages, but initial studies and reports from the field indicate that this is a promising approach (Dillon & Hornstein, 2013; Longden, Read, & Dillon, 2018) and may thus also have potential to support the deprescribing process when patients seek this out. It is perhaps premature for providers to recommend progressive approaches such as this, for example in schizophrenia, as an evidence-based alternative to gold standard care. Although participation can derive significant benefits for those inclined, potential risks must also be considered—including disincentivizing to avail of (other) evidence based treatments where indicated.

Alternatives to Suicide groups, developed by the Western Massachusetts Recovery Learning Community, provide spaces for people to talk openly about their thoughts and feelings about suicide. These are groups where discussions of suicide take place without a clinical staff member present, making open conversation possible without the potential of involuntary commitment (WMRLC, 2018). Another example of peer and mutual support, these group seem well-suited to supporting people interested in a deprescribing trial.

Conclusion

Addressing potential reemergence of symptoms is a key practice in deprescribing, especially as the anticipatory anxiety around this possibility is hypothesized to potentially precipitate the feared outcome. Preplanning tools such as a PAD, WRAP, or other personally identified strategies for catching and addressing early warning signs are perhaps most successful when done in close collaboration with treatment team members and other significant people in the patient's life. Also, family education and involvement can provide a further dimension of support. Patient-determined wellness strategies offer additional treatments to ameliorate specific symptoms, improve social supports, and enhance the potential for finding meaning and purpose during deprescribing.

Self-Assessment

1. Relapse in psychiatry is:
   a. Easily definably and measurable using biological markers
   b. Personally defined by the patient
   c. Marked by reduction in functioning

    d. Often defined by proxy using hospitalization as the marker

    e. A and b

    f. B and d

    g. B, c, and d

Correct answer: g

2. WRAP plans must be shared with the clinical team as part of the philosophy of the approach.

    a. True

    b. False

Correct answer: b

3. Personal medicine is defined by Pat Deegan as:

    a. Individualized dosing of psychotropic medications

    b. A sugar pill designed to elicit the placebo effect

    c. Personal nonpharmacological approaches such as exercise

    d. Medicine not legal in all 50 US states

Correct answer: c

References

Alvarez-Jimenez, M., Priede, A., Hetrick, S. E., Bendall, S., Killackey, E., Parker, A. G., . . . Gleeson, J. F. (2012). Risk factors for relapse following treatment for first episode psychosis: a systematic review and meta-analysis of longitudinal studies. *Schizophrenia research, 139*(1-3), 116–128.

Bandura, A. (1977). Self-efficacy: Toward a unifying theory of behavior change. *Psychological Reviews, 84*(2), 191–215.

Birchwood, M., Smith, J., Macmillan, F., Hogg, B., Prasad, R., Harvey, C., & Bering, S. (1989). Predicting relapse in schizophrenia: the development and implementation of an early signs monitoring system using patients and families as observers, a preliminary investigation. *Psychological Medicine, 19*(3), 649–656.

Butzlaff, R. L., & Hooley, J. M. (1998). Expressed emotion and psychiatric relapse: A meta-analysis. *Archives of General Psychiatry, 55*(6), 547–552. doi: 10.1001/archpsyc.55.6.547.

Cechnicki, A., Bielańska, A., Hanuszkiewicz, I., & Daren, A. (2013). The predictive validity of Expressed Emotions (EE) in schizophrenia. A 20-year prospective study. *Journal of Psychiatric Research*, *47*(2), 208–214. doi: http://dx.doi.org/10.1016/j.jpsychires.2012.10.004.

Cook, J. A., Copeland, M. E., Hamilton, M. M., Jonikas, J. A., Razzano, L. A., Floyd, C. B., . . . Grey, D. D. (2009). Initial outcomes of a mental illness self-management program based on wellness recovery action planning. *Psychiatric Services*, *60*(2), 246–249.

Cook, J. A., Copeland, M. E., Jonikas, J. A., Hamilton, M. M., Razzano, L. A., Grey, D. D., . . . Carter, T. M. (2011). Results of a randomized controlled trial of mental illness self-management using Wellness Recovery Action Planning. *Schizophrenia Bulletin*, *38*(4), 881–891.

Cooney, G., Dwan, K., & Mead, G. (2014). Exercise for depression. *JAMA*, *311*(23), 2432–2433. doi: 10.1001/jama.2014.4930.

Copeland, M. E. (1997). *Wellness Recovery Action Plan*. Dummerston, Vermont: Peachtree Press.

Corstens, D., Longden, E., McCarthy-Jones, S., Waddingham, R., & Thomas, N. (2014). Emerging perspectives from the Hearing Voices Movement: Implications for research and practice. *Schizophrenia Bulletin*, *40*(Suppl_4), S285–S294. doi: 10.1093/schbul/sbu007.

Dauwan, M., Begemann, M. J., Heringa, S. M., & Sommer, I. E. (2016). Exercise improves clinical symptoms, quality of life, global functioning, and depression in schizophrenia: A systematic review and meta-analysis. *Schizophrenia Bulletin*, *42*(3), 588–599. doi: 10.1093/schbul/sbv164.

DeBrul, S., & The Icarus Project. (2015). Mad maps. http://www.pdf-archive.com/2015/11/06/madnessandoppressionguide/. Accessed January 15, 2016.

Deegan, P. E. (2005). The importance of personal medicine: A qualitative study of resilience in people with psychiatric disabilities. *Scandinavian Journal of Public Health*, *33*(66_suppl), 29–35. doi: 10.1080/14034950510033345.

Deegan, P. E., Carpenter-Song, E., Drake, R. E., Naslund, J. A., Luciano, A., & Hutchison, S. L. (2017). Enhancing clients' communication regarding goals for using psychiatric medications. *Psychiatric Services*, *68*(8), 771–775. doi: 10.1176/appi.ps.201600418.

Dillon, J., & Hornstein, G. A. (2013). Hearing voices peer support groups: A powerful alternative for people in distress. *Psychosis*, *5*(3), 286–295. doi: 10.1080/17522439.2013.843020.

Dillon, J., & Longden, E. (2013). Hearing voices groups. In M. Romme & S. Escher, eds., *Psychosis as a personal crisis: An experience based approach*, UK: Routledge, 129–140.

Falloon, I. R. (2003). Family interventions for mental disorders: Efficacy and effectiveness. *World Psychiatry*, *2*(1), 20–28.

Firth, J., Cotter, J., Elliott, R., French, P., & Yung, A. R. (2015). A systematic review and meta-analysis of exercise interventions in schizophrenia patients. *Psychological Medicine, 45*(7), 1343–1361. doi: 10.1017/S0033291714003110.

Gorczynski, P., & Faulkner, G. (2010). Exercise therapy for schizophrenia. *Cochrane Database of Systematic Reviews* (5). doi: 10.1002/14651858. CD004412.pub2.

Greer, T. L., & Trivedi, M. H. (2009). Exercise in the treatment of depression. *Current Psychiatry Reports, 11*(6), 466. doi: 10.1007/s11920–009-0071–4.

Jamison, K. R. (1995). *An Unquiet Mind.* New York: Alfred A Knopf.

Knapen, J., Vancampfort, D., Moriën, Y., & Marchal, Y. (2015). Exercise therapy improves both mental and physical health in patients with major depression. *Disability and Rehabilitation, 37*(16), 1490–1495. doi: 10.3109/ 09638288.2014.972579.

Longden, E., Read, J., & Dillon, J. (2018). Assessing the impact and effectiveness of Hearing Voices Network self-help groups. *Community Mental Health Journal, 54*(2), 184–188. doi: 10.1007/s10597-017-0148-1.

Mackler, D., & Morrissey, M. (2010). *A Way Out of Madness: Dealing with Your Family After You've Been Diagnosed with a Psychiatric Disorder.* New York: AuthorHouse.

McFarlane, W. R. (2002). *Multifamily Groups in the Treatment of Severe Psychiatric Disorders.* New York: Guilford Press.

Oregon Behavioral HelathNetwork, (2016). Personal action/crisis prevention plan. https://www.mvbcn.org/wp-content/uploads/Crisis-Prevention-Plan-Adult-2017.pdf. Accessed April 3, 2019.

O'Connell, M. (2015). Psychiatric advance directives. In P. W. Corrigan (Ed.), *Person-Centered Care for Mental Illness: The Evolution of Adherence and Self-Determination* (pp. 103–116). Washington, DC: American Psychological Association.

Payne, T., Allen, J., & Lavender, T. (2017). Hearing Voices Network groups: Experiences of eight voice hearers and the connection to group processes and recovery. *Psychosis, 9*(3), 205–215. doi: 10.1080/ 17522439.2017.1300183

Pharoah, F., Mari, J., Rathbone, J., & Wong, W. (2010). Family intervention for schizophrenia. *The Cochrane Database of Systematic Reviews*(12), CD000088–CD000088. doi: 10.1002/14651858.CD000088.pub2.

Pilling, S., Bebbington, P., Kuipers, E., Garety, P., Geddes, J., Orbach, G., & Morgan, C. (2002). Psychological treatments in schizophrenia: I. Meta-analysis of family intervention and cognitive behaviour therapy. *Psychological Medicine, 32*(5), 763–782. doi: 10.1017/S0033291702005895.

Romme, M., Escher, S., Dillon, J., Corstens, D., & Morris, M. (2009). *Living with Voices: 50 Stories of Recovery*. Ross-on-Wye, UK: PCCS books.

Saks, E. R. (2007). *The Center Cannot Hold: My Journey Through Madness*. London: Hachette UK.

Scheewe, T. W., Backx, F. J. G., Takken, T., Jörg, F., van Strater, A. C. P., Kroes, A. G., . . . Cahn, W. (2013). Exercise therapy improves mental and physical health in schizophrenia: A randomised controlled trial. *Acta Psychiatrica Scandinavica, 127*(6), 464–473. doi: 10.1111/acps.12029.

Scott, A., & Wilson, L. (2011). Valued identities and deficit identities: Wellness Recovery Action Planning and self-management in mental health. *Nursing inquiry, 18*(1), 40–49.

State of Maine Substance Abuse and Mental Health Services. (2016). Rights and legal issues crisis planning. http://www.maine.gov/dhhs/samhs/mentalhealth/rights-legal/crisis-plan/home.html. Accessed January 15, 2016.

Styron, T., Utter, L., & Davidson, L. (2017). The hearing voices network: Initial lessons and future directions for mental health professionals and Systems of Care. *Psychiatry Quarterly*. doi: 10.1007/s11126-017-9491-1.

Swanson, J. W., Swartz, M. S., Elbogen, E. B., Van Dorn, R. A., Wagner, H. R., Moser, L. A., . . . Gilbert, A. R. (2008). Psychiatric advance directives and reduction of coercive crisis interventions. *Journal of Mental Health (Abingdon, England), 17*(3), 255–267. doi: 10.1080/09638230802052195.

Swarbrick, M. (2006). A wellness approach. *Psychiatric Rehabilitation Journal, 29*(4), 311–314.

WMRLC. (2018). Alternatives to suicide. http://www.westernmassrlc.org/alternatives-to-suicide. Accessed July 30, 2018.

Zika, S., & Chamberlain, K. (1992). On the relation between meaning in life and psychological well-being. *British Journal of Psychology, 83*(1), 133–145. doi: 10.1111/j.2044-8295.1992.tb02429.x.

6

Wellness Approaches II

Collaborative Strategies

When considering a course of deprescribing, in addition to the personal, self-determined strategies addressed in Chapter 5, it is essential to evaluate the person's interest in and potential benefit from specific modalities of psychotherapy, symptom support, and other clinical interventions. This chapter covers some of the more commonly used approaches as well as briefly discussing emerging and progressive practices. As in Chapter 5, we reiterate our advocacy, in general, for a multi-facted treatment approach considering multiple dimensions. In comparison to chapter 5, the evidence base for the effectiveness of some of the following strategies in certain conditions is more developed, however we again caution against using the promise of such interventions to justify a reactive abandonment of pharmacotherapy. We again encourage prescribers to actively discuss (if not deliver themselves) non-pharmacological treatment options to build alliance and allow the patient to integrate all facets of their treatment. Similar to Chapter 5 we also include a targeted review of the literature for the relatively uninitiated reader.

Goal and Learning Objectives

After reading this chapter, the reader will be able to:

1. Identify two evidence-based psychotherapies to consider adding during deprescribing
2. Identify two benefits of peer support
3. Describe the importance of sleep management as part of a deprescribing trial

Additional Clinical Strategies

Depending on the condition, several specific psychotherapies may be considered as adjunctive, or even primary, modalities of treatment to add when considering a course of deprescribing. In this section, we will describe several key therapies that may be useful adjuncts (e.g., CBT and Acceptance and Commitment Therapy), the importance of addressing sleep issues, and progressive and emerging approaches including online and mobile technologies.

Acceptance and Commitment Therapy

One evidence-based adjunctive psychotherapy that cuts across symptoms and conditions is *Acceptance and Commitment Therapy* (ACT, Hayes, Strosahl, & Wilson, 1999). Considered a third-wave cognitive therapy, it focuses on the pursuit of valued goals, the increase of psychological flexibility, detachment from language as fact, and use of mindfulness. ACT is considered an evidence-based practice (SAMHSA, 2010) and an approach to alleviating human distress and suffering with underlying mechanisms that are transdiagnostic (Hayes et al., 1999). Evidence for its use with obsessive compulsive disorder (OCD), depression, rehospitalization due to any reason, psychosis, and general mental health are validated by SAMHSA, although other clinical trials show promise for its use in chronic pain (see Powers, Zum Vorde Sive Vording, & Emmelkamp, 2009, for a meta-analysis) and voice hearing (Bach & Hayes, 2002; Gaudiano & Herbert, 2006). Growing evidence for its use with schizophrenia is emerging (Shawyer et al., 2017), but further trials are needed to confirm greater efficacy over the comparison condition of befriending. In serious mental illness, ACT can be integrated within a multi-dimensional treatment plan, including the consideration of pharmacotherapy.

ACT's grounding theory is not disorder-specific but is instead aimed at reducing suffering through experiential and mindfulness approaches, with a focus on values-based living, thus making it a promising treatment modality for people with a complex constellations of problems and in line with recovery-oriented approaches to care (Davidson, Rowe, Tondora, O'Connell, & Lawless, 2008; Tondora, Miller, Slade, & Davidson, 2014). ACT works to change one's relationship with distress, regardless of etiology, as opposed to necessarily trying to change thoughts or feelings. Instead, the focus is on *accepting* thoughts, feelings, and experiences and finding ways to still work toward valued life goals through increasing psychological flexibility (Ciarrochi, Bilich, & Godsell, 2010). ACT is one modality to consider adding for someone interested in initiating a course of deprescribing.

Cognitive Behavior Therapy

Traditional CBT has a strong evidence base in treating anxiety (Stewart & Chambless, 2009), depression (Cuijpers et al., 2013), OCD (Öst, Havnen, Hansen, & Kvale, 2015), and other conditions. A preliminary meta-analysis found that CBT for depression showed equivalent efficacy to pharmacotherapy, with long-term gains better maintained via CBT than medications (Gould, Otto, Pollack, & Yap, 1997). A recent meta-analysis looking at depression and anxiety disorders found combination therapy most effective, with both pharmacotherapy and behavioral interventions providing independent and long-lasting effects (Cuijpers et al., 2014). As an adjunct, CBT-informed treatments have also been shown in a recent meta-analysis to help prevent the transition into psychosis (Hutton & Taylor, 2014), and is a recommended treatment for schizophrenia as part of a multi-dimensional plan of care including pharmacotherapy (Dixon et al., 2009).

More recently, adjunctive CBT for psychosis (CBTp; Turkington & Kingdon, 1998) has shown positive results for those with psychotic experiences, however meta-analysis level evidence remains inconclusive. This modification of traditional CBT directly addresses positive and negative symptoms by widening coping strategies, reducing distress caused by voices or other positive symptoms, and increasing understanding of the problems in the person's life. It is goal-focused, meant to be collaborative, and is focused on improving quality of life. Therapist and client come to an understanding together of what is leading to the identified problems—and they come to a mutual formulation of such. It also involves evaluating the evidence for and against beliefs, including delusional ones, and indicating how likely these beliefs are true (Hagen, Turkington, Berge, & Gråwe, 2013; Turkington, Wright, & Tai, 2013). More recent iterations of CBTp have shifted to an even more strengths-based and values and goals focus, one consistent with recovery-oriented care (Anthony, 1993; Turkington et al., 2013). It remains likely that antipsychotics would continue to play a vital role in psychotic disorder treatment and towards the optimal delivery of CBTp, however combined strategies may help support minimum effective dosing.

Sleep

Patients may rightly fear the reemergence of sleep disturbances when starting a reduction of medications. One of the most significant predictors and risk factors in schizophrenia, mood disorders, and other psychiatric disorders is that of *sleep changes*. In a recent meta-analysis, people with schizophrenia who were not taking medications had significantly shorter total sleep time, sleep onset latency, and sleep efficiency, and those who had been withdrawn from medications had a similar profile for those three variables (Chan, Chung, Yung, & Yeung, 2017). Sleep changes have moderate predictive validity of relapse in psychotic disorders (Eisner, Drake, & Barrowclough, 2013).

Sleep disturbances in affective disorders has been well-documented, both via self-report and through objective study, and they carry an increased risk of suicidality (Rumble, White, & Benca, 2015). Relevant disturbances include shorter total sleep time, greater sleep onset latency, and decreased sleep efficiency. Sleep disturbance and insomnia have also been found to be independent predictors of depression (Rumble et al., 2015). Therefore, addressing sleep is a major focus area for deprescribing psychotropic medications overall and in particular for antipsychotic medications (Klingaman, Palmer-Bacon, Bennett, & Rowland, 2015), due to the common collateral sedative effects of these medications (Rumble et al., 2015).

Sleep disturbances have been found to have moderate predictive value in relapse for psychotic disorders (Eisner et al., 2013). In another review looking at predictors of relapse in schizophrenia, increased emotional sensitivity was found to be moderately predictive (Gaebel & Riesbeck, 2014), but overall there were few specific and sensitive signs that accurately predicted relapse. An increase in anxiety has also been identified as a moderate predictor of relapse (Eisner et al., 2013). One meta-analysis found that critical comments by caregivers (negative expressed emotions) increased the likelihood of relapse by 2.2 times in first-episode psychosis (Alvarez-Jimenez et al., 2012).

Sleep emerges as a particularly important focal point in a recent study of people discontinuing a range of psychiatric medications (Ostrow, Jessell, Hurd, Darrow, & Cohen, 2017). The first study of its kind, the research found that sleep was the most important factor in helping cope with potential withdrawal effects. Recent recommendations for treatment of sleep disturbances in general regard behavioral and psychological treatments as first-line and more effective long-term than pharmacological interventions (Morgenthaler et al., 2006; Morin, Culbert, & Schwartz, 1994). These treatments include CBT for insomnia (CBT-I), relaxation training, and stimulus control therapy (reassociating the bedroom with sleep), as well as using paradoxical intention (setting the goal as staying awake) to reduce performance anxiety (Morin et al., 1994). These treatments have also been found to be effective for those with co-occurring psychiatric disorders and insomnia (Taylor & Pruiksma, 2014). Treating other causes of sleep disturbance is also important, and patients should be assessed for sleep apnea or other obstructive disorders which can greatly impact sleep quality and duration. This is especially true for those patients on antipsychotic and other medications that might have contributed to the development of metabolic syndrome, with the associated weight gain contributing to sleep apnea (Rumble et al., 2015).

Peer Support

Peer support is another adjunctive support to consider in the process of deprescribing. Peer support is defined as "a system of giving and receiving help founded on key principles of respect, shared responsibility, and mutual agreement of what is helpful" (Mead, 2003). It is the provision of support from those with "lived experience" of mental illness and/or substance use disorders. As a growing field and discipline, research shows that outcomes from working with peer staff are equivalent to non-peer staff, with some studies showing slightly better outcomes with peer staff (Solomon, 1995; Davidson, 2004). Patients experienced longer community tenure when receiving peer support in one randomized controlled trial (Min 2007). Peer staff also show an ability to reach people who are difficult to engage (Rowe, 2007; Sells, 2006). Working with peers contributes to increases in empowerment (Corrigan, 2006; Resnick, 2008) and an increased sense of independence for both peer staff and the person receiving services, as well as role shift (Ochocka, 2006). Those patients working with peers also showed increased hope (Sledge, 2011). The overall evidence base for adjunctive peer support is considered moderate (Chinman, 2014). Peer support provides a unique opportunity to show that recovery is real through living examples.

Novel and Progressive Approaches

Behavioral management techniques can be used to cope with voices, including listening to music, distraction, physical exercise, and other techniques. Such strategies can be taught prior to or in the process of deprescribing, where appropriate, in order to build the repertoire of coping for the person experiencing (or fearing the experience of) distressing voices. The theory is that subjective fear as well as the actual risk of relapse are reduced (Deegan & Affa, 1995).

Towards normalization of patient experiences, one can potentially generalize the idea of redefining symptoms as "extreme states" to psychiatric hospitalization. As previously noted, relapse is often defined by hospitalization (Lader, 1995), but if we can work to destigmatize the idea of hospitalization as something that is less of a "failure" and characterize it more as another tool in the coterie of possible strategic ways to take care of oneself, perhaps better use can be made of our inpatient facilities. This may be a challenge for many patients because their hospital experiences may have been traumatic—another reason to work to avoid returning to the hospital. Use of alternatives to hospitalization (e.g., peer run respites, intensive outpatient services, and other crisis intervention residential services) may be options to identify ahead of time for when a person needs more support but not necessarily inpatient hospitalization.

Another progressive approach gaining recognition is *open dialogue*. Open dialogue is an approach developed in the mid 1990s in Finland using a multifaceted conversation to prevent relapse, particularly in first-episode psychosis (Seikkula, Alakare, & Aaltonen, 2001). The intervention begins within 24 hours of onset and includes bringing together the person's social network and providers in conversation. The intention is to provide words and description to the experience and to reconnect the person with those important others in their life (Seikkula et al., 2006). Several important principles of the approach include continuity of care, involvement of family and caregivers in dialogue together with the person, and tolerance of uncertainty as more important than change (Pavlovic, Pavlovic, & Donaldson, 2016). A recently published 19-year observational study from Finland showed that open dialogue reduced the need for neuroleptics and improved social and occupational outcomes (Bergström et al., 2018). However, a review of the evidence on open dialogue concluded that although it appears promising, the current evidence base in its support is of low quality and weak (Freeman, Tribe, Stott, & Pilling, 2018). Although open dialogue may offer some useful principles which, relevant to deprescribing, may have potential to support minimum effective dosing of medications, it cannot currently be recommended in place of gold standard treatments for psychotic disorders.

Online Resources and Apps for Therapy and Support

Increasingly, online resources and smartphone applications are being utilized for both therapy and adjunctive support of deprescribing and addressing particular symptoms. The Veteran's Affairs department has sponsored the development of several useful apps to supplement posttraumatic stress disorder (PTSD) treatment and CBT for insomnia treatment (Kuhn et al., 2016). An initial RCT for the CBT-I coach app for mobile phones found good acceptability and positive outcomes in veterans also enrolled in a CBT-I therapy (Koffel et al., 2018). Similar positive results for the PTSD Coach app have been found, with strong acceptability (Miner et al., 2016) and initial positive evaluation results (Kuhn et al., 2014; Owen et al., 2015). A recent RCT showed significant effects on PTSD and depressive and anxiety symptoms (Kuhn et al., 2017).

Internet-based CBT interventions have shown increasing promise across a range of symptoms and conditions in recent years. A meta-analysis of 19 RCTs showed support for clinical improvement in depression, with those interventions that provided additional supportive interventions having a greater effect size (Richards & Richardson, 2012). Guided therapies, those using the support of a therapist either in person or by phone, have shown greater effectiveness than those without. However even without this therapist interaction, internet-based interventions show a significant impact on depression, as analyzed in another review of 22 studies (Iakimova, Dimitrova, & Burté, 2017). A recent study comparing internet-based CBT to face-to-face delivered interventions showed no difference in overall effects, although there was a limited pool of studies to draw on, indicating more research needed in this area (Andersson, Cuijpers, Carlbring, Riper, & Hedman, 2014).

An ever-evolving array of wellness-related apps are becoming increasingly accessible, and these also leverage multiple modes of passive data collection/sensing built into mobile devices and wearable technology. While at the disposal of the interested and informed individual as tools to maintain wellness, the clinical effectiveness of these applications warrants rigorous ongoing study.

Conclusion

A brief summary of recommendations for supporting deprescribing using wellness strategies (drawn from the content of Chapters 5 and 6) is provided in Table 6.1. In short, individualizing and tailoring a patient's particular plan to his or her particular needs and concerns stands the best chance of preventing or foreshortening feared outcomes. For some people, there may not be a need to add any additional supports; this should be assessed very

Table 6.1 Identifying adjunctive wellness strategies to support deprescribing

Concern or area of need	Consider adding or recommending:
Clinical supports and specific symptoms	Cognitive behavioral therapy (ACT, CBT, CBTp) Sleep hygiene/CBTi Exercise Peer support/mutual support groups Using technology to supplement these supports
Concerns regarding relapse	Psychiatric Advance Directive (PAD) Wellness Recovery Action Plan (WRAP) Other preplanning tools Normalizing and decatastrophizing relapse and hospitalization Assessing level of fear via dialogue or use of FORSE
Social support	Family psychoeducation Family therapy Social skills or supported socialization Incorporating friends and acquaintances into the deprescribing plan
Meaning and purpose	Identifying interests, hobbies and values Referral to employment support Finding a job or starting volunteer work

ACT, acceptance and commitment therapy; CBT, cognitive behavior therapy; CBTb, cognitive behavior theory for psychosis; CBTi, cognitive behavior theory for insomnia; FORSE, fear of recurrence scale.

carefully and with the consideration that adding supports may also signal a concern on the part of the prescriber to the patient regarding their worry or level of confidence in the deprescribing process. Similar caution should be taken in making recommendation of non-evidence based strategies—or at least providing clear caveats and limitations when drawing a patient's attention to a progressive or self-directed strategy. If not framed in a balanced way, the process of introducing alternatives to pharmacotherapy risks having these novel, non-threatening and compelling strategies over-valued, at least beyond their current evidence base. In this way therapeutic alliance may be weakened, rather than strengthened. Therefore, acknowledging the potential usefulness and eliciting the patient's own preferences is an important step in conveying confidence in the ability of the patient to embark on the deprescribing process, but our expertise and value as prescribers (and deprescribers) should not be relinquished. At the same time, it is important to look closely at possible additional supports that will decrease the likelihood of a negative impact of a reduction in medications.

Overall these additional supports should be seen in the context of empowering the person to find new ways of supporting their recovery and learning strategies for managing symptoms, or, put more colloquially, *live the life that they want to live without (or with a reduction of) medications.* Framing the whole deprescribing intervention in these terms is important (and not just lip service) as it promotes a certain responsibility and interdependence in the person. Learned helplessness, dependency, and lack of trust in oneself are some of the possible relics of the paternalistic approach to prescribing medications, and being aware of these dynamics is essential in thinking about "prescribing" other interventions for the person.

Self-Assessment

1. **One of the key symptoms to address in order to help prevent relapse is:**
   a. Auditory hallucinations
   b. Anxiety around the deprescribing process
   c. OCD-like symptoms that emerge within the discontinuation process
   d. Lack of sleep/insomnia
   Correct answer: D

2. You are working with a 45-year-old woman who has a 15-year history of schizoaffective disorder and is interested in decreasing her haloperidol and sertraline due to feelings of sedation and emotional dulling. She is currently living alone in her apartment and tends to come out only to see you for monthly appointments. Which of the following would you recommend to her to support her interest in deprescribing?
   a. Completing a values survey to identify what is most important to her and start with the first ranked value
   b. Refer her to the local psychosocial clubhouse to get more friends
   c. Refer her to employment support so she can begin looking for a job
   d. Discuss a range of options and elicit her thoughts, values, and preferences, utilizing a shared decision-making approach
   Correct answer: D

3. Acceptance and Commitment therapy is focused on:
   a. Changing negative thoughts to positive ones
   b. Identifying cognitive distortions
   c. Increasing psychological flexibility
   d. Pinpointing core beliefs
   Correct answer: C

References

Alvarez-Jimenez, M., Priede, A., Hetrick, S. E., Bendall, S., Killackey, E., Parker, A. G., . . . Gleeson, J. F. (2012). Risk factors for relapse following treatment for first episode psychosis: A systematic review and meta-analysis of longitudinal studies. *Schizophrenia Research, 139*(1–3), 116–128. doi: https://doi.org/10.1016/j.schres.2012.05.007.

Andersson, G., Cuijpers, P., Carlbring, P., Riper, H., & Hedman, E. (2014). Guided Internet-based vs. face-to-face cognitive behavior therapy for psychiatric and somatic disorders: A systematic review and meta-analysis. *World Psychiatry, 13*(3), 288–295.

Anthony, W. A. (1993). Recovery from mental illness: The guiding vision of the mental health service system in the 1990s. *Psychosocial Rehabilitation Journal, 16*(4), 11.

Bach, P., & Hayes, S. C. (2002). The use of acceptance and commitment therapy to prevent the rehospitalization of psychotic patients: A randomized controlled trial. *Journal Consulting and Clinical Psychology, 70*(5), 1129–1139.

Bergström, T., Seikkula, J., Alakare, B., Mäki, P., Köngäs-Saviaro, P., Taskila, J. J., . . . Aaltonen, J. (2018). The family-oriented open dialogue approach in the treatment of first-episode psychosis: Nineteen-year outcomes. *Psychiatry Research, 270*, 168–175.

Chan, M.-S., Chung, K.-F., Yung, K.-P., & Yeung, W.-F. (2017). Sleep in schizophrenia: A systematic review and meta-analysis of polysomnographic findings in case-control studies. *Sleep Medicine Reviews, 32*, 69–84. doi: https://doi.org/10.1016/j.smrv.2016.03.001.

Chinman, M., George, P., Dougherty, R. H., Daniels, A. S., Ghose, S. S., Swift, A., & Delphin-Rittmon, M. E. (2014). Peer support services for individuals with serious mental illnesses: Assessing the evidence. *Psychiatric Services, 65*(4), 429–441. doi: 10.1176/appi.ps.201300244

Ciarrochi, J., Bilich, L., & Godsell, C. (2010). Psychological flexibility as a mechanism of change in acceptance and commitment therapy. In R. Baer, ed., *Assessing mindfulness and acceptance processes in clients: Illuminating the theory and practice of change.* New Harbinger: Oakland, CA, pp. 51–75.

Corrigan, P. W. (2006). Impact of consumer-operated services on empowerment and recovery of people with psychiatric disabilities. *Psychiatric Services, 57*(10), 1493–1496.

Cuijpers, P., Berking, M., Andersson, G., Quigley, L., Kleiboer, A., & Dobson, K. S. (2013). A meta-analysis of cognitive-behavioural therapy for adult depression, alone and in comparison with other treatments. *The Canadian Journal of Psychiatry, 58*(7), 376–385. doi: 10.1177/070674371305800702.

Cuijpers, P., Sijbrandij, M., Koole, S. L., Andersson, G., Beekman, A. T., & Reynolds, C. F. (2014). Adding psychotherapy to antidepressant medication in depression and anxiety disorders: A meta-analysis. *World Psychiatry, 13*(1), 56–67.

Davidson, L., Shahar, G., Stayner, D. A., Chinman, M. J., Rakfeldt, J., & Tebes, J. K. (2004). Supported socialization for people with psychiatric disabilities: Lessons from a randomized controlled trial. *Journal of Community Psychology, 32*(4), 453–477.

Davidson, L., Rowe, M., Tondora, J., O'Connell, M. J., & Lawless, M. S. (2008). *A Practical Guide to Recovery-Oriented Practice: Tools for Transforming Mental Health Care.* New York: Oxford University Press.

Deegan, P. E., & Affa, C. (1995). *Coping with Voices: Self Help Strategies for People Who Hear Voices That Are Distressing.* National Empowerment Center.

Dixon, L. B., Dickerson, F., Bellack, A. S., Bennett, M., Dickinson, D., Goldberg, R. W., . . . Pasillas, R. M. (2009). The 2009 schizophrenia PORT psychosocial treatment recommendations and summary statements. *Schizophrenia Bulletin, 36*(1), 48–70.

Eisner, E., Drake, R., & Barrowclough, C. (2013). Assessing early signs of relapse in psychosis: Review and future directions. *Clinical Psychology Review, 33*(5), 637–653. doi: http://dx.doi.org/10.1016/j.cpr.2013.04.001.

Freeman, A. M., Tribe, R. H., Stott, J. C., & Pilling, S. (2018). Open dialogue: A review of the evidence. *Psychiatric Services, 70*(1), 46–59.

Gaebel, W., & Riesbeck, M. (2014). Are there clinically useful predictors and early warning signs for pending relapse? *Schizophrenia Research, 152*(2–3), 469–477. doi: https://doi.org/10.1016/j.schres.2013.08.003.

Gaudiano, B. A., & Herbert, J. D. (2006). Acute treatment of inpatients with psychotic symptoms using Acceptance and Commitment Therapy: Pilot results. *Behavioral Research and Therapy, 44*(3), 415–437. doi: 10.1016/j.brat.2005.02.007.

Gould, R. A., Otto, M. W., Pollack, M. H., & Yap, L. (1997). Cognitive behavioral and pharmacological treatment of generalized anxiety disorder: A preliminary meta-analysis. *Behavior Therapy, 28*(2), 285–305.

Hagen, R., Turkington, D., Berge, T., & Gråwe, R. W. (2013). *CBT for Psychosis: A Symptom-Based Approach*. New York: Routledge.

Hayes, S. C., Strosahl, K. D., & Wilson, K. G. (1999). *Acceptance and Commitment Therapy: An Experiential Approach to Behavior Change*. New York: Guilford.

Hutton, P., & Taylor, P. J. (2014). Cognitive behavioural therapy for psychosis prevention: A systematic review and meta-analysis. *Psychological Medicine, 44*(3), 449–468.

Iakimova, G., Dimitrova, S., & Burté, T. (2017). Can we do therapy without a therapist? Active components of computer-based CBT for depression. *L'Encephale, 43*(6), 582–593.

Klingaman, E. A., Palmer-Bacon, J., Bennett, M. E., & Rowland, L. M. (2015). Sleep disorders among people with schizophrenia: Emerging research. *Current Psychiatry Reports, 17*(10), 79. doi: 10.1007/s11920-015-0616-7.

Koffel, E., Kuhn, E., Petsoulis, N., Erbes, C. R., Anders, S., Hoffman, J. E., . . . Polusny, M. A. (2018). A randomized controlled pilot study of CBT-I Coach: Feasibility, acceptability, and potential impact of a mobile phone application for patients in cognitive behavioral therapy for insomnia. *Health Informatics Journal, 24*(1), 3–13.

Kuhn, E., Greene, C., Hoffman, J., Nguyen, T., Wald, L., Schmidt, J., . . . Ruzek, J. (2014). Preliminary evaluation of PTSD Coach, a smartphone app for post-traumatic stress symptoms. *Military Medicine, 179*(1), 12–18.

Kuhn, E., Kanuri, N., Hoffman, J. E., Garvert, D. W., Ruzek, J. I., & Taylor, C. B. (2017). A randomized controlled trial of a smartphone app for posttraumatic stress disorder symptoms. *Journal of Consulting and Clinical Psychology, 85*(3), 267.

Kuhn, E., Weiss, B. J., Taylor, K. L., Hoffman, J. E., Ramsey, K. M., Manber, R., . . . Trockel, M. (2016). CBT-I coach: A description and clinician perceptions of a mobile app for cognitive behavioral therapy for insomnia. *Journal of Clinical Sleep Medicine, 12*(04), 597–606.

Lader, M. (1995). What is relapse in schizophrenia? *International Clinical Psychopharmacology, 9*, 5–10.

Mead, S. (2003). Defining peer support. *Intentional peer support: An alternative approach.* www.intentionalpeersupport.org. Accessed June 5, 2017.

Min, S.-Y., Whitecraft, J., Rothbard, A. B., & Salzer, M. S. (2007). Peer support for persons with co-occurring disorders and community tenure: A survival analysis. *Psychiatric Rehabilitation Journal, 30*(3), 207–213. doi: 10.2975/30.3.2007.207.213

Miner, A., Kuhn, E., Hoffman, J. E., Owen, J. E., Ruzek, J. I., & Taylor, C. B. (2016). Feasibility, acceptability, and potential efficacy of the PTSD Coach app: A pilot randomized controlled trial with community trauma survivors. *Psychological Trauma, 8*(3), 384.

Morgenthaler, T., Kramer, M., Alessi, C., Friedman, L., Boehlecke, B., Brown, T., . . . Owens, J. (2006). Practice parameters for the psychological and behavioral treatment of insomnia: An update. An American Academy of Sleep Medicine report. *Sleep, 29*(11), 1415.

Morin, C. M., Culbert, J. P., & Schwartz, S. M. (1994). Nonpharmacological interventions for insomnia. *American Journal of Psychiatry, 151*(8), 1172.

Ochocka, J., Nelson, G., Janzen, R., & Trainor, J. (2006). A longitudinal study of mental health consumer/survivor initiatives: Part 3—A qualitative study of impacts of participation on new members. *Journal of Community Psychology, 34*(3), 273–283.

Öst, L.-G., Havnen, A., Hansen, B., & Kvale, G. (2015). Cognitive behavioral treatments of obsessive–compulsive disorder. A systematic review and meta-analysis of studies published 1993–2014. *Clinical Psychology Review, 40*, 156–169.

Ostrow, L., Jessell, L., Hurd, M., Darrow, S. M., & Cohen, D. (2017). Discontinuing psychiatric medications: A survey of long-term users.

Psychiatric Services, *68*(12), 1232–1238. appi.ps.201700070. doi: 10.1176/appi.ps.201700070.

Owen, J. E., Jaworski, B. K., Kuhn, E., Makin-Byrd, K. N., Ramsey, K. M., & Hoffman, J. E. (2015). mHealth in the wild: Using novel data to examine the reach, use, and impact of PTSD coach. *JMIR Mental Health*, *2*(1), e7.

Pavlovic, R. Y., Pavlovic, A., & Donaldson, S. (2016). Open Dialogue for psychosis or severe mental illness. *Cochrane Database of Systematic Reviews*(10). doi: 10.1002/14651858.CD012384.

Powers, M. B., Zum Vorde Sive Vording, M. B., & Emmelkamp, P. M. (2009). Acceptance and commitment therapy: A meta-analytic review. *Psychotherapy and Psychosomatics*, *78*(2), 73–80. doi: 10.1159/000190790.

Resnick, S. G., & Rosenheck, R. A. (2008). Integrating peer-provided services: a quasi-experimental study of recovery orientation, confidence, and empowerment. *Psychiatric Services*, *59*(11), 1307–1314.

Richards, D., & Richardson, T. (2012). Computer-based psychological treatments for depression: A systematic review and meta-analysis. *Clinical Psychology Review*, *32*(4), 329–342. doi: https://doi.org/10.1016/j.cpr.2012.02.004.

Rowe, M., Bellamy, C., Baranoski, M., Wieland, M., O'connell, M. J., Benedict, P., . . . Sells, D. (2007). A peer-support, group intervention to reduce substance use and criminality among persons with severe mental illness. *Psychiatric Services*, *58*(7), 955–961.

Rumble, M. E., White, K. H., & Benca, R. M. (2015). Sleep disturbances in mood disorders. *Psychiatric Clinics of North America*, *38*(4), 743–759. doi: http://dx.doi.org/10.1016/j.psc.2015.07.006.

SAMHSA. (2010). Acceptance and commitment therapy. http://legacy.nreppadmin.net/ViewIntervention.aspx?id=191. Accessed July 19, 2017.

Seikkula, J., Aaltonen, J., Alakare, B., Haarakangas, K., Keränen, J., & Lehtinen, K. (2006). Five-year experience of first-episode nonaffective psychosis in open-dialogue approach: Treatment principles, follow-up outcomes, and two case studies. *Psychotherapy Research*, *16*(2), 214–228. doi: 10.1080/10503300500268490.

Seikkula, J., Alakare, B., & Aaltonen, J. (2001). Open dialogue in psychosis I: An introduction and case illustration. *Journal of Constructivist Psychology*, *14*(4), 247–265. doi: 10.1080/10720530125965.

Sells, D., Davidson, L., Jewell, C., Falzer, P., & Rowe, M. (2006). The treatment relationship in peer-based and regular case management for clients with severe mental illness. *Psychiatric Services*, *57*(8), 1179–1184.

Shawyer, F., Farhall, J., Thomas, N., Hayes, S. C., Gallop, R., Copolov, D., & Castle, D. J. (2017). Acceptance and commitment therapy for psychosis: Randomised controlled trial. *British Journal of Psychiatry*, *210*(2), 140–148. doi: 10.1192/bjp.bp.116.182865.

Sledge, W. H., Lawless, M., Sells, D., Wieland, M., O'Connell, M. J., & Davidson, L. (2011). Effectiveness of peer support in reducing readmissions of persons with multiple psychiatric hospitalizations. *Psychiatric Services*, *62*(5), 541–544.

Solomon, P., & Draine, J. (1995). One-year outcomes of a randomized clinical trial of consumer case management. *Evaluation and Program Planning*, *18*(2), 117–127

Stewart, R. E., & Chambless, D. L. (2009). Cognitive–behavioral therapy for adult anxiety disorders in clinical practice: A meta-analysis of effectiveness studies. *Journal of Consulting and Clinical Psychology*, *77*(4), 595.

Taylor, D. J., & Pruiksma, K. E. (2014). Cognitive and behavioural therapy for insomnia (CBT-I) in psychiatric populations: A systematic review. *International Review of Psychiatry*, *26*(2), 205–213.

Tondora, J., Miller, R., Slade, M., & Davidson, L. (2014). *Partnering for Recovery in Mental Health: A Practical Guide to Person-Centered Planning*. New York: John Wiley & Sons.

Turkington, D., & Kingdon, D. (1998). CBT for psychosis *Outcome and Innovation in Psychological Treatments of Schizophrenia*. Chichester, UK: John Wiley & Sons.

Turkington, D., Wright, N. P., & Tai, S. (2013). Advances in cognitive behavior therapy for psychosis. *International Journal of Cognitive Therapy*, *6*(2), 150–170.

7

The Process of Deprescribing

Minimum effective dosing and discontinuation of psychiatric medications are neither new nor foreign concepts. "Deprescribing," however, as a relatively recently coined term, could represent several advancements for psychiatry as: (1) a rallying call to the field to more concertedly examine the factors that influence and inform our prescribing both on an individual and system levels; (2) an expanding area of research seeking answers to questions around medication reduction and guidance for interested prescribers; and (3) perhaps most importantly, a structured, multi-facted intervention for optimizing the collaborative and concerted reduction of a chosen medication.

Goal and Learning Objectives

After reading this chapter, the reader will be able to:

1. Identify three scenarios in one's past or current practice where deprescribing might be considered
2. Define and differentiate a paternalistic, consumerist and shared decision-making stance as they might pertain to deprescribing
3. Outline the seven steps of deprescribing in psychiatry

Deprescribing as an intervention is much more than a trial of discontinuation or withdrawal of medications. Its development as an intervention has so far been led by pharmacists (see Farrell et al., 2015; Reeve, Thompson, & Farrell, 2017). Reeve and colleagues (2014) reviewed the available literature on the deprescribing process and identified five essential key elements. Of note, only one is the actual discontinuation. These elements are:

1. Obtaining a complete medication history.
2. Identifying medications that are potentially inappropriate.

3. Evaluating the possibility of reducing and/or discontinuing the medication.
4. Implementing a plan for reducing and/or discontinuing the medication.
5. Ongoing monitoring, documentation and support.

When attempting to adapt this work, which has principally thus far in primary care and geriatric and palliative medicine, to psychiatry, we propose some additional considerations. These are by no means unique to mental health, but perhaps more salient because of previously discussed sociocultural and individual factors which have a particular impact in the practice of psychiatry. These include:

- A greater focus on the therapeutic alliance and the psycho-sociocultural context
- The risk of faddism, pendulum-swinging, and the unintentional creation of stigma
- The broader context and timing of the intervention
- Opportunities for leveraging nonpharmacologic strategies and treatments
- The psychodynamic meaning of the medication (and diagnosis)
- Managing the illusion of diagnostic and therapeutic precision
- Tolerance of uncertainty and ambiguity
- Working within legally mandated treatment stipulations
- Broadening the group of stakeholders involved
- Scenarios in which a patient's capacity is impacted or a surrogate decision-maker is appointed
- Limitations and realities of current resources (e.g., scope and duration of appointment or access to nonpharmacological treatments)

In light of these additional considerations for deprescribing in psychiatry, we have therefore expanded Reeve's five steps to seven. We have added these steps in order to reflect an extended preparatory phase which puts additional focus on the timing of the intervention, inclusion of significant social supports, and bolstering of psychosocial and clinical supports that clinical experience indicates are essential to safely reducing and discontinuing psychotropic medications (Gupta & Cahill, 2016). These additional steps reflect the multidimensional nature of recovery and provide an opportunity to explore and bolster the therapeutic relationship and plan of care as well as empower the patient. In fact, we propose that this phase may stand alone as a valuable exercise even if it does not immediately or ever lead to a plan to alter a person's medication regimen. The proposed seven steps of deprescribing in psychiatry, split into a "preparation" and an "action" phase (in respect to medication dosing), are described in Table 7.1. For each step, the main, intended *aims* and *outcomes* are listed to offer a starting point for the practitioner.

Table 7.1 Proposed steps for deprescribing in psychiatry

Step	Aims	Outcomes
Preparation phase		
1 **Assess the timing and context**	• Be planful to optimize chances of success • Remain alert to periods of, and factors driving, higher risk of relapse • Reinforce that deprescribing is an option (if not now, in the future)	• Detailed bio-psych-social-cultural assessment with focus on factors known to drive relapse • Gain alliance around disclosure and monitoring of substance use • Anticipate stressors (next 6 months) • Proceed now or postpone for later date
2 **Medication reconciliation**	• Compile a detailed list of all current medications (from all providers) • Include alternative remedies • Elicit specific, underdisclosed side effects (e.g., sexual, check renal function) • Facilitate the patient articulating associated pros and cons of taking each medication • Acknowledge (and communicate acceptance) that conflict and ambivalence around treatment is expected	• A complete list of all medications taken • An opportunity for further psychoeducation • Gain and document permission to communicate with other prescribers • Gain access to relevant medical records • Develop a common appreciation and language around the ongoing benefits and risks of each medication • Uncover ambivalence and actual level of adherence • Reveal undisclosed experiences/side effects

(continued)

Table 7.1 Continued

Step	Aims	Outcomes
3 *Explore patient's experience, attitudes and meaning around treatment*	• Explore the patient's thoughts and feelings around their condition and its treatment as a whole • Detect potential nonpharmacological effects of medications (i.e., meaning-based) • Explore experience of existing treatments and previous attempts at deprescribing	• An opportunity to bolster therapeutic alliance and empower patient • Learn patient's learning style preference and assessment of current understanding • Appreciate patient's frame of reference and core values relevant to treatment decisions • Consider with patient whether to proceed to action phase now, or cycle back to Step 1 at later date
Action phase		
4 *Set frame for the deprescribing intervention*	• Discuss with patient possible outcomes (including adverse outcomes/relapse) • Elicit their hopes, ideas, concerns and expectation for the process • Have patient identify key supports and treaters they wish to involve in process • Demonstrate interest, optimism and expertise in the process	• Gain informed consent around next phase of the intervention • Engage and secure two-way line of communication with key supports • Understand how patient likes to make decisions • Gain mutual respect for each other's expertise/ experience
5 *Decide which medication to deprescribe*	• Exam benefits and risks of deprescribing up to three medications (involve key supports as needed) • Provide decision support tools to patient as desired and useful • Engage in shared decision making to choose 1 to deprescribe now	• Document shared decision-making process • Agree upon medication to deprescribe (may take several meetings) • Further develop therapeutic alliance and a spirit of collaborative investigation (within safe bounds)

Table 7.1 Continued

Step	Aims	Outcomes
6 *Develop the specific deprescribing plan*	• Identify established and new nonpharmacological treatments and strategies to treat emergent effects of reduction and maintain wellness • Set clear expectations and action plan, including wellness/crisis planning • Identify early warning signs of relapse • Use existing clinical evidence/experience to plan rate of taper and identify pharmacological strategies for emergent effects (i.e., short-term adjunctive drugs)	• Document expected and possible effects with guidelines for responding to each • Construct a detailed step-by-step dose reduction plan with schedule of monitoring • Share a copy with key supports • Confirm understanding of deprescribing plan • Ensure full access to necessary, expanded nonpharmacological treatments and wellness strategies • Engender broad buy-in and optimism around plan among key stakeholders
7 *Implement, monitor and adjust plan (according to response)*	• Implement changes and monitoring according to plan • Remain open to need for adjusting the plan • Monitor mental and physical status • Monitor occupational and social functioning • Loop back to Step 6 as necessary • Be able to accept failure of the intervention without reproach	• Deprescribing may be completed as planned • May need to adjust (e.g., slow the rate of, or reverse the taper) • May need to manage a relapse/adverse event • Patient hopefully gains a deeper understanding of themselves and empowered management of their condition (whatever the outcomes) • Therapeutic alliance and treatment is enriched and knowledge is gained (and ideally shared)

As mentioned, the initial preparation phase can stand alone as a periodic medication review process, perhaps done every 6 months or annually whether or not it leads to a formal deprescribing of a chosen medication. The intervention proper begins in the second "action" phase with Step

4. A deprescribing effort may be initiated by the patient, prescriber, or another stakeholder. One of the aspirational, collateral benefits of this deprescribing intervention (specifically the preparation phase) is to illuminate and normalize previously undisclosed ambivalence and 'true adherence' to current prescribed medication regimens. Taking this further, and in order to avoid precipitous, patient-initiated discontinuations, we recommend that, as part of the process of *prescribing*, providers also consider setting parameters and expectations around the option of *deprescribing*. Deprescribing may therefore be more than just a tool to be used as the circumstance arises.

There are potential risks as well as benefits with deprescribing as with any other intervention, and informed consent is paramount. To truly engage our patients in shared decision-making we also potentially engage them in shared risk-taking. It remains the duty of each provider to weigh the balance of evidence in any individual case when deciding whether or not to recommend deprescribing. This includes remaining reflective and observant of their practice (and that of their immediate colleagues), as well as staying up to date with the clinical evidence and guidelines. However, it is not and should not be the sole responsibility of the prescriber to initiate, gather additional information and resources, and "manage" a deprescribing process.

Step 1: Assess the Timing and Context

This stage is predicated on having an up-to-date, bio-psycho-social-cultural formulation, medical, and psychiatric assessment as well as a strong therapeutic alliance. It is crucial to develop an open line of communication around substance use, whether it be direct disclosure from the patient or indirect via periodic urine toxicology if warranted by a recent history of substance use disorder. Although current use of substances would not automatically preclude deprescribing, it is best to have a clear sense of the current use of substances, and to be thinking of past use as a potential risk factor for the person, who may turn to restarting or increasing substances in response to a decrease in prescribed medications.

Stress commonly exacerbates many psychiatric disorders (Lex, Bäzner, & Meyer, 2017). Though impossible to anticipate all potential psychosocial stressors, there are circumstances that the patient and/or therapist may assume will be stressful, such as a change in employment, housing, relationships, therapist, or psychiatrist. An attempt at medication reduction would be least risky when the patient has a relatively stable psychosocial situation. For example, the immediate posthospitalization period is known to carry higher clinical risk and planned medication reductions should be implemented cautiously (Olfson et al., 2016). Well-intentioned prescribers may need to carefully balance the need for postdischarge dose reductions, which, although they may be clearly warranted after acute stabilization, other psychosocial circumstances may point to waiting before beginning deprescribing. This may be when collateral tranquilizing effects are no longer needed, psychosocial factors have improved, or simply due to the natural course of the illness episode.

Medication reduction may be easier and safer in a patient who is able to gauge their emotional state and communicate either directly with the prescriber or through family and friends. Past experiences with a patient around life events and the demonstrated ability of the patient to reach out for additional support from treaters and others, is a positive sign for this ability to be used during deprescribing. The use of tracking tools such as symptom scales or daily recording of moods, etc., can be useful in this area. At the same time, a patient who is less able to identify and clearly report changes should not be excluded from consideration, particularly if there is a clear rationale (e.g., metabolic syndrome, sedation) that more clearly points to deprescribing as an important intervention in mitigating risk. Impending significant life events or logistical barriers should be planned around (e.g., moving or a transition to college). The prescriber will need to thoroughly evaluate past responses to medication reduction and evaluate risk (past attempts at suicide, homicide, legal involvement) in considering deprescribing for a given patient. The outcome of this step may be to postpone the deprescribing until later while reinforcing that it is an option and laying any necessary groundwork in the meantime (e.g., treat an active substance use disorder).

Step 2: Medication Reconciliation

The major outcomes of this step are a complete and detailed list of medications that the client is currently taking, access to appropriate records and providers, and gaining a deeper appreciation of the individual effects of each medication for the patient. This may likely include uncovering ambivalence or actual adherence to the prescribed regimen around certain medications or dosages—which should be met with acceptance and understanding. This step will likely require liaison with the primary care provider and other specialists. Ask explicitly about nonprescription, over-the-counter medications; medications used on an as-needed basis; additional doses taken outside of how the medication was prescribed; and alternative, natural, and traditional remedies (in order to consider potential pharmacologic or nonpharmacologic effects and interactions). The list should ideally describe each medication in a manner identifiable to the patient—strength and dosage form, for example "20 mg enteric-coated tablet" may be paired with "small white pill with 57 on it." The list should also be assessed for possible drug–drug interactions, additive side effects, and disease–drug interactions (ideally in collaboration with a pharmacist and informed by the patient's latest health status).

It can be challenging to deduce the original therapeutic target or intent when a medication (and dose) was initiated by a prior provider—it cannot be assumed that the medication was prescribed for the principal US Food and Drug Administration (FDA)-approved indication, for example. The original indication for a medication may not be clearly documented and may require extensive record-searching (Plakiotis et al., 2015; Reeve et al., 2014; Scott et al., 2015). Real-world practice dispels the illusion of therapeutic precision; for example, a change in prescriber may interrupt plans for cross-titration of antipsychotic medications or discontinuation of an anticholinergic during antipsychotic titration, thus leading to inadvertent and irrational polypharmacy. Similarly, an antipsychotic initiated at higher doses for the treatment of acute mania with psychotic features and severe agitation during an inpatient admission, if unexamined, may cloud the clinical picture either by implying the definitive diagnosis of a primary psychotic disorder or causing secondary negative symptoms.

Once the list is compiled, conduct a systematic reexamination of the pros and cons of *continuing* each medication at all, and at its current respective dose. It is advisable to neither constrain this discussion to what the prescriber would consider conventional therapeutic and adverse effects, nor be too exhaustive in listing all the rarer potential side effects per package insert or case report-level evidence—as always, the process should be tailored to the patient according to good clinical judgment. Thus, for the prescriber, this step provides an opportunity to learn and reconcile an individual patient's experience with a given medication (perhaps even idiosyncratic beliefs) with their existing knowledge base.

Step 3: Explore Patient's Experience, Attitudes, and Meaning About Medication

A patient's experience of a medication is his or her own. Effects of the idiosyncratic "meaning" of a medication can present consciously and unconsciously. Furthermore, attitudes toward taking or not taking medications may vary with culture, personality, and specific relationship with the prescriber (Jonsdottir et al., 2013; Lanouette, Folsom, Sciolla, & Jeste, 2015; Misdrahi et al., 2012; Sylvia et al., 2013). In the same way that providers offer their perspectives on etiology and mechanisms of action (invited or not), it is valuable to gain an understanding of the patient's perspective on the source of their distress and how they maintain their wellness. This can lead to useful elucidation of the concepts of symptom management, *diagnosis, prognosis*, and phases of illness/recovery.

Power struggles and transference-based issues may manifest in discussions surrounding medication (Mallo & Mintz, 2013), and the prescriber should maintain a psychotherapeutically informed stance within the scope of their training and treatment frame while exploring these issues. Collaboration with a patient's therapist may help. As discussed in Chapter 6, medication may hold psychodynamic meaning for a patient (e.g., representing the prior treater who originally prescribed it and thus representing a symbolic loss of the relationship to give it up), be viewed as a "badge of illness" (e.g., evidence of a medical explanation for their struggles), or as vital to their accessing resources (notably entitlements).

The outcome of Step 3 (and hence the preparation phase) of deprescribing may equally be the decision to cycle back around at a later date than to proceed with a deprescribing trial—but it should always result in a deepening of the patient's understanding, empowerment, and ownership of their recovery and the treatment relationship.

Step 4: Set the Frame for the Deprescribing Intervention

Step 4 begins the "action phase" of the deprescribing intervention proper and therefore should begin with a process of informed consent. Solicit patient preferences on receiving and manipulating information (i.e., verbal, written, or digital) and who they would like to include in the decision-making process. Provide an overview of deprescribing as a potential treatment direction in order to solicit ideas, concerns, and expectations from the patient, their family, and even the clinical care team. It is important to acknowledge the potential risks (including adverse outcomes, symptom increase, and relapse) as well as differentiating these risks in the context of a slow process of deprescribing with increased attention in contrast to unsupported or even precipitous medication discontinuations.

The patient may receive pressure and mixed messages from their key supports around their interest in deprescribing. This can contribute to stress and undermine an attempt at deprescribing; therefore, it is the responsibility of the prescriber to identify these supports and assist the patient to engage with and involve them at their comfort level. Expectation of a relapse or a negative outcome can actually increase the possibility of a negative outcome and hence it is especially important to elicit potential concerns from the patient and their key supports and to address all possible (Colloca & Finniss, 2012). Despite these challenges it is possible to generate buy-in, optimism, and enthusiasm for a deprescribing process, so long as realistic expectations are set, concerns are addressed, and opportunities for meaningful growth through collaborative inquiry are well-articulated.

Step 5: Decide Which Medication to Deprescribe

This step involves a concerted, shared decision-making process. While acknowledging the potential for differing opinions on which medication should be deprescribed (e.g., the prescriber might prioritize a reduction in the benzodiazepine, but the patient might elect to start with the antipsychotic), we suggest limiting the medications discussed in detail at this stage to no more than three. Systematically weigh together in greater detail the risks and benefits, this time, of *deprescribing* each option (this inversion from Step 2, may yield further and confirm previously acquired data). Specifically raise adverse effects that may be initially asymptomatic (such as early chronic renal impairment); tend to be underreported (such as sexual side effects); or can be associated with lesser subjective distress than functional impact (such as tardive dyskinesia). The principal outcome of this step is agreement around a single medication to be deprescribed—this may be an important exercise in balancing power dynamics in the therapeutic relationship and might raise ethical issues. As stated earlier, shared decision-making is neither paternalism nor consumerism, and both patient and prescriber should have their voices present in the room. It may be helpful to consider more diffuse or downstream therapeutic gains in addition to the specifics of the task in hand. The prescriber might seek peer supervision or local ethics committee consultation in acknowledging how challenging—but meaningful—this process can be.

Step 6: Develop the Specific Deprescribing Plan

The foundations of a good deprescribing plan include setting clear expectations, bolstering alternative coping and wellness strategies, and fostering an acceptance of the inherent uncertainty of the process. The deprescribing plan therefore draws on the best available clinical evidence and knowledge of and from the individual patient to determine a "good enough" initial rate of taper, establish a robust safety net for emergent effects and burgeoning relapse, and a clear rationale for attempting the deprescribing regardless of the eventual outcome. The chosen medication may be tapered to a new target, gradually discontinued, or, perhaps in other cases, switched to an alternative with more favorable side-effect profile but lesser expected efficacy.

The deprescribing plan should integrate features and language specific to the individual patient and context, pitched at an appropriate level of education and insight. Psychotropic medications can produce distressing withdrawal symptoms (Dilsaver & Alessi, 1988; Tamam & Ozpoyraz, 2002; Wyatt, 1991), and it is important to generate realistic expectations, assess for them at every visit, and offer in advance, management strategies. This may take the form of wellness recovery action planning (WRAP; Copeland, 1997); a psychiatric advance directive or other preplanning tools described in Chapter 6; or our Collaborative Deprescribing Worksheet (proposed below). Specify new and existing alternative treatments as well as early warning signs of relapse, using the patient's own words (reflecting together on the time course of prior episodes of illness may be useful in this respect). Additionally, deprescribing studies in geriatric medicine suggest a role for family (Plakiotis et al., 2015), and interventions such as family therapy and relapse prevention strategies may be beneficial (Emslie et al., 2015; Hasan & Musleh, 2017; Pitschel-Walz, Leucht, Bäuml, Kissling, & Engel, 2015). Wellness strategies should draw from the patient's own ideas and methods (even if initially regarded by the provider as idiosyncratic). There may be further opportunity here to reconcile countertherapeutic behaviors with available clinical evidence. Wellness strategies may be collaborative (with supports or providers) or be self-directed (in which case, they may not be discussed in detail or at all with the prescriber).

More frequent clinical encounters and/or the provision for additional ad hoc sessions may be planned (within the limitations of available resources and the patient's schedule). Providers should remain mindful, make good use of their own reactions, and recognize the potential for altering the frame (i.e., duration and frequency of visits) based on countertransference (e.g., increased contact due to unfounded anxiety, or diminished contact due to discomfort sitting with emerging symptoms, loss of control, or increased risk).

Step 7: Implement, Monitor, and Adjust Plan

It is crucial for both prescriber and patient to be flexible and view medication changes as "trials" (Reeve et al., 2014) that can be adjusted as needed. Once again, framing the patient's recovery as a complex system, and deprescribing as a complex intervention, this process can be regarded as "probing and monitoring response," or "safe to fail" collaborative inquiry. As for safety, a measured and feasible crisis plan should have been well-articulated in Step 6, setting the bounds within which adaptations to the plan would be acceptable in Step 7. Modifications may include slowing of the taper; introducing a short-term, as-needed medication for emerging symptoms; or even re-titrating the medication and reassessing.

Periodic monitoring of all aspects of a patient's health and functioning is indicated, with particular focus on the anticipated effects. Both prescriber and patient take joint responsibility in this plan. In all cases, fostering a stance of optimism and acceptance in the patient and the potential outcomes is key. Ensure that the patient remains empowered in process, is utilizing their strengths, and is deriving the intended benefit from new and supplemental strategies and supports. As part of the monitoring process, providers should also consider the meaning of the deprescribing intervention itself to the patient and to themselves, meanings which can shift and evolve. For example, overinvestment (e.g., due to a patient's desire to please the prescriber) may extend a deprescribing past a shift in the risk–benefit ratio. Alternatively, intolerance of anxiety or a residual difference in opinion on which medication to deprescribe might drive the premature abandonment of an otherwise potentially successful discontinuation.

Documentation of Deprescribing

Accurate documentation of a deprescribing intervention is essential for several reasons. Because deprescribing may not adhere to standard guidelines, documenting clear rationales and plans may help allay any potential medico-legal issues. Furthermore, the patient–prescriber team may need to repeatedly refer to a plan during the process. Finally, because guidelines and published clinical evidence are currently lacking, a detailed case history (used locally or published) may help accumulate knowledge and guide deprescribing interventions for other patients. The structure of the clinical instrument we in this chapter below (if with the proper consent, appropriately de-identified and incorporated into a suitable platform) may serve as a means of recording and sharing the process and events of deprescribing towards generating a database for continuous learning and innovation (akin to a Learning Health System).

Electronic medical records, progress notes, or medication order forms are typically not set up for the documentation of process and are meant mainly for recording of observations, diagnoses, and orders. We recommend a more holistic documentation of medication lists, with due attention being paid to the understanding and value that the patient attaches to each of the medications. Box 7.1 shows an example of such a medication list. Collateral information on the effects of specific interventions applied can additionally add context and guide the deprescribing.

The authors offer the reader a collaborative deprescribing worksheet (Appendix 1). This document is designed to be completed and maintained by both the patient and prescriber as a framework to help guide, promote, and document a person-centered collaborative deprescribing process (it should not be overvalued as the core intervention in and of itself). There are three parts, which can be used independently or together as one document: Part A documents information gathering and sharing, Part B documents a shared decision-making process, and Part C documents details and implementation of the deprescribing plan (while allowing for

Box 7.1 Example Format for Collaboratively Documenting Medication Lists

Patient's name: *John Smith*

Date: *10/20/2018*

Sources of information: *John and his wife (Tina), pharmacy, psychiatric records, primary care records*

Participants: *John and Tina, therapist (via phone)*

Medication and dose	Started on	Clinical Indication for medication	Side effects	Patient/caregiver Perceived usefulness
Depakote 1,000 mg BID	Apr 2008	Mood stabilization	Hair loss	John thinks it is "useless." Tina thinks John gets angry if he misses morning doses.
Risperidone 4 mg HS	Apr 2008	Psychotic symptoms	None	Both John and Tina agree that risperidone keeps him "even."
Cogentin 2 mg HS	Jun 2008	Risperidone-induced EPS	None	"Don't know." "Haven't taken it at times."
Wellbutrin 400 mg daily	May 2011	Depressive symptoms in the context of bereavement	None	"Really helped back then." Therapist thinks it helped him quit smoking.
Protonix 40 mg daily	Jan 2012	Heartburn	None	"I can't stop this one. I get chest pain without it."
Lipitor 80 mg at bedtime	Jan 2018	High cholesterol	None	"The doc said I need it to keep my cholesterol down."

flexibility). The patient and prescriber are both invited to sign their names on this document to reflect the collaborative nature of the process. The authors encourage practitioners to consider adopting the worksheet as is, or adapting it to their needs. A digital version can be readily developed and integrated into electronic medical records.

Part A: *Reviewing the medications*

In Part A, the patient and prescriber gain a shared understanding of *all* current medications taken (this may include alternative remedies if relevant). Collaborate on listing both the current and potentially future "pros versus cons" of taking each medication in commonly understood language. These may include pertinent positive and negative effects as well as other factors like cost and convenience that emerge from your discussion. Potential side effects should be curated to those most relevant (avoid simply listing all possible associated side effects of each medication). You should extend into further rows of the worksheet (and an additional side) if needed. As you work through, flag up to three medications that either patient or prescriber wishes to consider further together for deprescribing. As mentioned earlier, a prescriber and patient may undertake Part A periodically, whether or not intending it to lead to a deprescribing. Part A encompasses the previously detailed deprescribing Steps 1 through 3.

Part B: *Choosing a medication*

In Part B, the patient and prescriber (soliciting additional input from key supports and additional resources as appropriate) engage in shared decision-making around which medication to deprescribe at this time. First, the patient identifies what factors/values are most important to them when making this decision (responding to the four direct questions). The patient's ideas, concerns, and expectations are elicited. The provider may assist the patient in identifying who else might be appropriate to involve in the deprescribing decision process—this may include key supports, peers, other providers, or consultants (such as pharmacists or other specialists). Once these foundations are in place, up to three medications (as identified in Part A) are examined in detail, asking the question: What are the potential benefits and risks of *deprescribing* the medication? Please note that, by contrast, in Part A the pros and cons of *continuing* each medication are examined. Part B refers to deprescribing Steps 4 and 5 and similarly concludes with the definitive agreement on one medication to deprescribe.

Part C: *The deprescribing plan*

In Part C, the specifics of the deprescribing plan are articulated, implemented, monitored, and adjusted as necessary. The workflow references the field of management's Plan-Do-Study-Act construct to capture the complexity of the process, the importance of starting somewhere, and learning and adapting, as well as balancing inherent elements of certainty and uncertainty. Expectations around anticipated emergent effects (such e.g., as insomnia) as the taper ensues are listed, with suggestions (from the prescriber, patient, and key supports) of what to try in response. This can include pharmacologic as well as nonpharmacologic strategies (such as, e.g., short-term use of a hypnotic agent, sleep hygiene practices, or cognitive behavior therapy). The prescriber also has the opportunity to stipulate scenarios in which they would like to be updated or consulted. Although taking a more directive stance here, this can be well-pitched to communicate an ongoing interest and concern for the patient, a "leaning in" and offering of a clear safety net. Similarly, circumstances that would constitute an emergency are listed. The log section offers a rolling audit trail of clinical events, which might include dose decrements, initiation of alternative treatments, or follow-up contacts. The patient has the opportunity to document any changes they notice at these time points and what strategies they employed in response, all of which will be available for discussion at the next review. At the end of each subsequent clinical encounter, the event log may be updated with agreed recommendations (and a copy made to chart). On a point of practicality, if plans need to be changed and a series of proposed actions are not implemented, they might be negated (with a single line) and the series continued in the row beneath from that point. Part C refers to deprescribing Steps 6 and 7.

Conclusion

This chapter has described an expanded process for deprescribing specifically adapted to psychiatry. The considerations and strategies are humbly offered serve as a starting point for the interested prescriber and what we hope will remain a burgeoning field. The principal addition to existing guidelines is a preparation phase that gathers further information on the wider context of the medication regimen and lays firm foundations for the intervention proper. As a complex intervention for a set of complex problems (which mental health conditions invariably represent), a commensurate approach finds a "good enough" starting point, probes and monitors closely (with multiple, iterative "safe to fail" trials), and accepts uncertainty while maintaining optimism. These principles may be equally relevant in treating an individual patient and in innovating in the field as a whole.

Self-Assessment

- Identify 3 cases from your past of present practice where deprescribing might have been/be relevant.
- With a colleague, role play the completion of the 7 steps of deprescribing using the instrument provided.
- Provide and receive feedback on how it felt in both roles (patient and prescriber), what went well, and what could be improved. Pay particular attention to dynamic shifts along the "continuum of shared decision-making".

References

Colloca, L., & Finniss, D. (2012). Nocebo effects, patient-clinician communication, and therapeutic outcomes. *JAMA, 307*(6), 567–568.

Copeland, M. E. (1997). *Wellness Recovery Action Plan.* Dummerston, Vermont: Peachtree Press.

Dilsaver, S., & Alessi, N. (1988). Antipsychotic withdrawal symptoms: Phenomenology and pathophysiology. *Acta Psychiatrica Scandinavica, 77*(3), 241–246.

Emslie, G. J., Kennard, B. D., Mayes, T. L., Nakonezny, P. A., Moore, J., Jones, J. M., . . . King, J. (2015). Continued effectiveness of relapse prevention cognitive-behavioral therapy following fluoxetine treatment in youth with major depressive disorder. *Journal of the American Academy of Child & Adolescent Psychiatry, 54*(12), 991–998.

Farrell, B., Tsang, C., Raman-Wilms, L., Irving, H., Conklin, J., & Pottie, K. (2015). What are priorities for deprescribing for elderly patients? Capturing the voice of practitioners: A modified delphi process. *PloS One, 10*(4), e0122246.

Gupta, S., & Cahill, J. D. (2016). A prescription for "deprescribing" in psychiatry. *Psychiatric Services, 14*(1), 4–11.

Hasan, A., & Musleh, M. (2017). The impact of an empowerment intervention on people with schizophrenia: Results of a randomized controlled trial. *International Journal of Social Psychiatry, 63*(3), 212–223. doi: 10.1177/0020764017693652.

Jonsdottir, H., Opjordsmoen, S., Birkenaes, A., Simonsen, C., Engh, J., Ringen, P., . . . Andreassen, O. (2013). Predictors of medication adherence in patients with schizophrenia and bipolar disorder. *Acta Psychiatrica Scandinavica*, *127*(1), 23–33.

Lanouette, N. M., Folsom, D. P., Sciolla, A., & Jeste, D. V. (2015). Psychotropic medication nonadherence among United States Latinos: A comprehensive literature review. *Psychiatric Services*, *60*(2), 157–174.

Lex, C., Bäzner, E., & Meyer, T. D. (2017). Does stress play a significant role in bipolar disorder? A meta-analysis. *Journal of Affective Disorders*, *208*, 298–308.

Mallo, C. J., & Mintz, D. L. (2013). Teaching all the evidence bases: Reintegrating psychodynamic aspects of prescribing into psychopharmacology training. *Psychodynamic Psychiatry*, *41*(1), 13.

Misdrahi, D., Petit, M., Blanc, O., Bayle, F., & Llorca, P.-M. (2012). The influence of therapeutic alliance and insight on medication adherence in schizophrenia. *Nordic Journal of Psychiatry*, *66*(1), 49–54.

Pitschel-Walz, G., Leucht, S., Bäuml, J., Kissling, W., & Engel, R. R. (2001). The effect of family interventions on relapse and rehospitalization in schizophrenia: A meta-analysis. *Schizophrenia Bulletin*, *67*(1), 73–92.

Plakiotis, C., Bell, J. S., Jeon, Y.-H., Pond, D., & O'Connor, D. W. (2015). Deprescribing psychotropic medications in aged care facilities: The potential role of family members. In P. Vlamos, A. Alexiou, eds., *GeNeDis 2014 2015* (pp. 29–43): Geneva, Switzerland: Springer.

Reeve, E., Shakib, S., Hendrix, I., Roberts, M. S., & Wiese, M. D. (2014). Review of deprescribing processes and development of an evidence-based, patient-centred deprescribing process. *British Journal of Clinical Pharmacology*, *78*(4), 738–747.

Reeve, E., Thompson, W., & Farrell, B. (2017). Deprescribing: A narrative review of the evidence and practical recommendations for recognizing opportunities and taking action. *European Journal of Internal Medicine*, *38*, 3–11. doi: http://dx.doi.org/10.1016/j.ejim.2016.12.021.

Scott, I. A., Hilmer, S. N., Reeve, E., Potter, K., Le Couteur, D., Rigby, D., ... Page, A. (2015). Reducing inappropriate polypharmacy: The process of deprescribing. *JAMA Internal Medicine*, *175*(5), 827–834.

Sylvia, L. G., Hay, A., Ostacher, M. J., Miklowitz, D. J., Nierenberg, A. A., Thase, M. E., . . . Perlis, R. H. (2013). Association between therapeutic alliance, care satisfaction, and pharmacological adherence in bipolar disorder. *Journal of Clinical Psychopharmacology*, *33*(3), 343–350.

Tamam, L., & Ozpoyraz, N. (2002). Selective serotonin reuptake inhibitor discontinuation syndrome: A review. *Advances in Therapy*, *19*(1), 17–26.

Wyatt, R. J. (1991). Neuroleptics and the natural course of schizophrenia. *Schizophrenia Bulletin*, *17*(2), 325.

8

Deprescribing Antidepressant Medications in Major Depressive Disorder

In this chapter, we discuss specific context, considerations and clinical decision-making relevant to deprescribing antidepressants. As in the subsequent medication class- and condition- specific chapters, we feel it justified to orient around both the available clinical efficacy and effectiveness literature, as well as what is (in our experience), real-world clinical practice and usage. Elsewhere, we raise possible alternative interpretations of established findings in order to remind the reader of the potential for subjectivity when drawing clinical inference from certain study designs. As stated previously, we propose that it is what the field at large holds true, not the raw sum of the clinical literature, that has greatest impact on real-world patient outcomes. We nevertheless trust that the reader will consider the literature and this work through their own critical lens of knowledge, experience and expertise. We include here proven, as well as hypothesized, potential adverse effects of extended AD use to promote inquiry by the individual prescriber and the field. Further, we discuss the clinical presentation and management of antidepressant discontinuation syndromes which may be encountered. Finally, we integrate pharmacological and non-pharmacological strategies that may support deprescribing ADs.

Goal and Learning Objectives

After reading this chapter, the reader will be able to:

1. Outline a framework for risk–benefit calculation for ongoing prescriptions of ADs
2. List common signs and symptoms of AD discontinuation syndrome and their management
3. Feel more empowered in developing an AD deprescribing plan for a given clinical scenario

Case Example

Joan is a 50-year-old woman who has had three episodes of depression and has been doing well on sertraline 100 mg/d for the past 3 years. She recently came across a newspaper article that questioned the efficacy of antidepressant medications and says that she may want to try stopping sertraline and managing any depressive symptoms through exercise and yoga. She brings this up with her prescriber at their next session. The prescriber advises that standard guidelines recommend indefinite continuation of maintenance treatment following three episodes of major depression, and that if Joan is interested in attempting to discontinue them, alternative strategies should be planned. Joan's prescriber choses to validate, that in addition to her personal preference here to not take ADs, growing numbers of reanalyses of data have questioned the efficacy of ADs for moderate depression. Before the tapering of sertraline is started, Joan realizes the need to consolidate her engagement in psychotherapy and making positive lifestyle changes (such as ensuring optimal sleep, diet and exercise, or minimizing unwarranted sources of stress in her environment). Education is provided about potential discontinuation symptoms, including the chances of feeling like she is experiencing a recurrence of depression. Other strategies for managing discontinuation symptoms, such as reducing the rate of taper, or a cross-taper to fluoxetine, are framed as potential options if necessary. Joan opts to start yoga and join a gym, and she and her prescriber decide to plan to start the taper in 1 month's time.

As debate questioning the use of antidepressants increasingly pervades public consciousness, psychiatric and primary providers may find themselves facing situations like Joan's with increasing frequency. ADs are a very commonly prescribed class of medication and are the first line treatment for most anxiety and depressive disorders, whilst being an adjunct for other conditions. It is particularly important to learn how to deprescribe ADs, firstly, because of how commonly they are prescribed and, secondly, because there *are* viable, evidence-based, nonpharmacological treatment alternatives in many situations. This chapter is intended to provide an approach to addressing such clinical scenarios. Table 8.1 lists the more commonly prescribed antidepressants and their indications.

Table 8.1 Commonly used antidepressant (AD) medications

Medication class	Common medications	Common indications
SSRIs	Fluoxetine, paroxetine, sertraline, citalopram, escitalopram, fluvoxamine	Depressive disorders, anxiety disorders, OCD, eating disorders, enuresis, neuralgia, migraines, smoking cessation
Tricyclic ADs	Imipramine, amitriptyline, nortriptyline, desipramine	
SNRIs	Venlafaxine, duloxetine	
Others	Bupropion, mirtazapine	

OCD, obsessive compulsive disorder; SNRI, selective serotonin norepinephrine inhibitors; SSRI, selective serotonin reuptake inhibitor.

Potential Effects of Extended Use of Antidepressants

Weight Gain

ADs belonging to the class monoamine oxidase inhibitors (MAOIs) and tricyclic antidepressants (TCAs) may contribute to weight gain both in the short- and long-term. Selective serotonin reuptake inhibitors (SSRIs), in contrast, vary in their effect on weight; fluoxetine and paroxetine are more often associated with the potential for weight loss, whereas citalopram and sertraline are thought of having lesser weight gain effects. Among the newer ADs, mirtazapine is widely associated with weight gain (often used an intended collateral effect), most of which occurs in the first 4 weeks. This topic is reviewed in more detail in the article by Fava (2000).

Sexual Dysfunction

ADs generally (excluding bupropion and mirtazapine) carry risk of causing a range of sexual side effects, including reduced libido, difficulty in arousal, erectile and ejaculatory dysfunction, and anorgasmia. Particularly problematic is the relative reluctance (potentially from both patient and provider) to raise the issue and the conflation or misattribution of effects being from the illness itself. Sexual side effects in turn can negatively affect a person's self-esteem, quality of life, and relationship with a partner.

Tardive or Withdrawal Dysphoria

Although not a well-established or accepted syndrome, it has been hypothesized that prolonged use or abrupt withdrawal of an AD can itself induce dysphoria. Equivalent phenomena are more established in antipsychotic treatment with the examples of tardive and withdrawal dyskinesia. To further explore the idea of tardive dysphoria, El-Mallakh et al. (2011) conducted a systematic review of existing long-term studies of AD treatment of recurrent depression. They concluded that while there was reliable evidence for AD efficacy in treatment of depressive episodes and preventing relapses of the same episode, the evidence for prevention of recurrences was less clear. Could some of the observed recurrences with AD maintenance represent tardive dysphoria?

El-Mallakh et al. (2011) identified 18 studies whose duration was more than 18 months and found that patients taking placebo were more likely to have recurrence of depression as compare to those taking ADs. However, results indicated that most of these recurrences occurred within the first 6 months of discontinuating, raising the possibility that AD withdrawal was responsible for the recurrence rather than the underlying disorder itself.

AD Tachyphylaxis or "Poop Out"

The reappearance of depressive symptoms when an AD is taken for maintenance, has been reported in some samples in over half of patients initially responding to an AD. This phenomenon (or group of phenomena) has been framed by some as AD tachyphylaxis or others, colloquially as "poop out". Some candidate mechanisms speculated to explain these clinical observations include a loss of placebo effect, pharmacokinetic changes, change in disease severity or pathogenesis, and ineffective prophylaxis. One question raised here is the whether the pathogenesis of a recurrence in a patient taking ADs is different from a person who has never taken an AD (see Byrne & Rothschild, 1998). Further research is needed in this area to better understand the relative contribution of underlying illness and medication effects to these scenarios.

Antidepressant Prescription in Primary Care

Primary care providers effectively screen for and manage a large proportion of major depressive disorder. ADs are prescribed commonly in primary care settings but unfortunately may be initiated and continued inappropriately (Baumeister, 2012). Primary care providers may only consider referring patients to specialist psychiatric providers if symptoms do not respond to a first or second trial of an AD, or striking behavioral side effects emerge (such as apparent activation of suicidality or mania). Without the support and input of specialists, recommendations for discontinuation may not be made and even when made, may not be followed as written. For instance, in a study targeting inappropriate AD prescription in primary care settings (e.g., using an AD for several years after remission of a single episode of major depression), it was found that only 6% of patients who were subsequently advised to discontinue their AD actually successfully followed through with the recommendation (Eveleigh et al., 2017). This study has important implications; first, when indicated, expectations for deprescribing should be established at the time of prescription (possibly with the input of specialists). Second, it suggests that AD discontinuation is not a simple matter of making a recommendation to discontinue a medication, and points to the need for the development and dissemination of complex, multi-faceted deprescribing interventions. Important for further research in this area is an exploration of the reasons behind the low percentage of follow through on the patient's part, which would further inform recommended interventions that might be particular to the primary care setting.

Relapse and Recurrence Prevention: The Role of ADs

In recurrent depressive disorder, a *relapse* is defined as the reappearance of depressive symptoms within the same episode of depression, whereas a *recurrence* is defined as the occurrence of a new episode of depression (Frank et al., 1991). Accordingly, continuation therapy with ADs would prevent relapse whereas maintenance therapy would prevent a recurrence. The Collaborative National Institute of Mental Health (NIMH) study recommended 16–20 weeks of continuation therapy based on the rationale that ADs merely suppress symptoms of a depressive episode rather than shortening its natural duration. Hence, treatment is needed for the entire natural duration of an episode, 6–8 weeks of acute treatment followed by 16–20 weeks of continuation; take for example work by Prien & Kupfer (1986). This study found that 38% of individuals assigned to placebo treatment in the continuation phase of treatment (after remission of acute symptoms with active treatment) relapsed as compared to 5% patients who were assigned to treatment with imipramine. However, notably, the AD used in the acute phase was discontinued abruptly with no washout period, risking a discontinuation syndrome and subsequent unblinding. Interestingly, rates of relapse for the placebo group and the imipramine group became almost equal after a further 8 weeks.

An extensive review of maintenance therapy with AD stated that "far fewer data exist on maintenance therapy and recurrence than is commonly thought" (Keller & Boland, 1998). The same review also concluded that maintenance therapy was recommended for anyone who had more than three episodes of depression, that tapering an AD was preferred to abrupt discontinuation, and that, although unexplored, psychotherapy was a promising intervention for prevention of recurrences. Since the publication of this review, there have been several longer term (varying between 1 and 5 years) trials of the efficacy of ADs, various psychotherapy modalities, and combinations thereof. However, reviews indicate that the average duration of trials still continues to center around 1 year (see Clarke, Mayo-Wilson, Kenny, & Pilling, 2015; Geddes et al., 2003).

Finally, in a recent commentary, Fava has raised the notion of a reconceptualization of some depressive recurrences as iatrogenic (secondary to AD treatment) and recommends a sequential model of treatment where the use of ADs is limited to the shortest period of time and then followed by the use of alternate strategies (Fava, 2018).

Risk of Recurrence

While considering deprescribing an AD, it is important to make a reasonable estimate of the risk for a recurrence of depression. If the risk for recurrence is high and the past episodes have been severe and disruptive to the patient's life, this needs to be weighed carefully. Contextualizing this is important, including looking at the patient's values regarding the use of psychotropic medications, the reported efficacy of the AD in preventing depressive recurrences, and the availability of alternate strategies for prevention of recurrences, as well as the person's willingness and access to these strategies.

Berwian and colleagues (2017) conducted a systematic review of 13 studies that identified predictors of a depressive relapse after AD discontinuation. They concluded that there was some evidence that the number of previous episodes and a true treatment response could predict a depressive relapse but that there was a critical need for further research in this area.

Planning Deprescribing of Antidepressants

After considering the risks of recurrence, side effects, patient preferences, and alternative maintenance treatments, the patient and prescriber may decide to attempt deprescribing. In planning AD deprescribing, as listed in Box 8.1, it is important to consider withdrawal symptoms and their management and the implementation of psychotherapeutic and behavioral interventions for prevention of recurrences.

Figure 8.1 lists key factors one may need to consider before making a decision about deprescribing ADs.

Box 8.1 Major Steps Involved in Deprescribing Antidepressant (AD) Medications

---

- Weigh risks of recurrence, efficacy of AD, side effects, availability of alternatives and patient preferences.
- Initiate psychotherapy and behavioral measures before AD reduction.
- Monitor factors that may increase a risk for recurrence (e.g. substance use or stress)
- Educate about, monitor, and manage AD withdrawal symptoms.

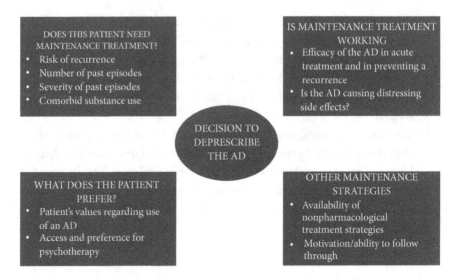

Figure 8.1 Some factors influencing the decision to deprescribe antidepressant medication in major depressive disorder.

Antidepressant Discontinuation or Withdrawal Syndromes

Although ADs have never been termed addictive and do not strictly meet criteria for such, discontinuation or withdrawal syndromes have been characterized. It is important to recognize and manage these transient symptoms of withdrawal as they can be misconstrued as a recurrence of the underlying depressive illness. In addition, the symptoms of withdrawal are reported as ranging from mild to very distressing to the patient. Numerous authors have reviewed clinical manifestations, mechanisms, and management strategies (see Haddad, 2001; Lejoyeux, Adès, Mourad, Solomon, & Dilsaver, 1996; Warner, Bobo, Warner, Reid, & Rachal, 2006). We have summarized the most relevant clinical information here.

Clinical Symptoms

Withdrawal symptoms have been described with all classes of serotonergic ADs including MAOIs, TCAs, SSRIs, and newer ADs such as the selective serotonin norepinephrine inhibitors (SNRIs) and noradrenergic and specific serotonergic antidepressants (NASSAs). Some withdrawal symptoms occurring after the abrupt discontinuation of tricyclic ADs however, have been attributed to a cholinergic rebound and have been treated with anticholinergic medications (see Dilsaver, Feinberg, & Greden, 1983). Symptoms of SSRI withdrawal are characteristic of the group and an *SSRI discontinuation syndrome* has been specifically named and described (estimated to occur in a third of individuals abruptly stopping). It is characterized by dizziness, fatigue, myalgia, paraesthesias, nausea, and vomiting (see Chouinard & Chouinard, 2015; Therrien & Markowitz, 1997). Mirtazapine withdrawal can cause a range of symptoms including insomnia, restlessness, nausea, vomiting, dizziness, agitation, panic attacks, mood swings, irritability, mania, or depression. These symptoms have been treated symptomatically with olanzapine, clonazepam, or fluoxetine depending on the presentation (see Cosci, 2017). Among SNRIs, venlafaxine has been shown to cause electric shock–like sensations similar to those described by patients withdrawing from SSRIs (see Reeves, Mack, & Beddingfield, 2003). In a study that pooled data from 553 patients, discontinuation of duloxetine was seen to most commonly cause dizziness, nausea, headache, and paraesthesia (Perahia, Kajdasz, Desaiah, & Haddad, 2005).

Variables Affecting Withdrawal Symptoms

Half-life, duration of treatment, dosage, and drug-drug interactions are to be considered when assessing likelihood of withdrawal symptoms. The *half-life* of the AD influences the likelihood of a patient developing withdrawal symptoms following AD discontinuation. ADs such as venlafaxine and paroxetine that have a half-life of less than 12 hours are more likely to cause withdrawal syndromes than fluoxetine, which has a half-life lasting days. ADs are unlikely to cause withdrawal if the *duration of treatment* was less than 5 weeks. Broadly, this may be reflective of intracellular changes induced by or adaptive to ADs over these initial weeks which become unopposed when the AD is abruptly removed. It is unclear if the *dose of the AD* influences the withdrawal symptoms. Additionally, there is some evidence to suggest that concurrent treatment with antihypertensives, anticonvulsants, and antihistamines is associated with a greater frequency of AD withdrawal symptoms (see Lejoyeux & Adès, 1997). Therefore, taking each of these variables into consideration is important when looking at rate of taper in ADs.

Differentiating withdrawal from a relapse or recurrence is important, as the management and prognosis of each differs, but clearly distinguishing each presents challenges. Antidepressant withdrawal typically begins a few days after the discontinuation of the medication and may be accompanied by numerous physical symptoms in addition to mood disturbances. Although a relapse may occur within a few days to weeks after AD discontinuation, it typically does not present with the physical symptoms characteristic of withdrawal syndromes. The distinction between AD withdrawal and major depressive relapse/recurrence may hold a different significance if some recurrences are indeed reformulated as being a function of AD use (see Fava, 2018). Adding to the conundrum of distinguishing the two (recurrence and withdrawal) is the common occurrence of patients skipping doses or taking brief 'holidays' from the medication. This can further muddy the picture, especially if the patient does not fully share the extent to which they have not adhered to the prescribed regimen.

An additional variable in depression treatment and subsequent AD withdrawal is hormonal variations and their effects on mood for women. Some pre-clinical evidence points to differential response to classes of ADs based on progesterone levels (Li et al., 2012). Also to be considered is stage of life (i.e., pre- peri- or post-menopausal) and relative contributions of the menstrual cycle on hormone and mood fluxuations. Although beyond the scope of this text, we encourage the reader to consider these as additional variables requiring consideration in the consideration of withdrawal symptoms and the differentiation between recurrence and withdrawal.

Managing AD Withdrawal

Unexpected and unmanaged withdrawal symptoms could easily prompt the abandoning of a deprescribing plan. Some of the most common strategies to address these symptoms include reducing the rate of taper of the AD or switching to long-acting agents such as fluoxetine. Consumer forums (uncontrolled, testimonial evidence) have described ways to take smaller doses of medication than are commercially available by crushing tablets or removing the contents of capsules to create smaller doses. Most recently, AD 'withdrawal strips' allow the patient to control the dosing in much smaller progressive decrements. Liquid preparations of many ADs are also available, but are not as commonly prescribed. Such extended taper strategies have been shown to reduce the incidence of withdrawal symptoms (see

Groot & van Os, 2018). However, the judicious reader should use caution in interpreting these mixed levels of evidence when attempting to infer the potential benefits and risks of this approach. Although is could be argued that both physiological and psychological aspects could be at play, a person-centered approach that accounts for non-pharmacological effects of medications (such as 'meaning') would accept value from so-called placebo effects. Further research in this area is much needed.

Psychotherapeutic and Behavioral Interventions to Support AD Deprescribing

Numerous psychotherapeutic approaches have shown efficacy in both the treatment of interepisodic residual symptoms and in the prevention of relapses and recurrences of major depression (see Nierenberg, Petersen, & Alpert, 2003). Psychotherapeutic interventions may very well become the mainstay of maintenance therapy in recurrent depression, especially if evidence for the iatrogenic theory of depression recurrence grows (see Fava, 2018).

Cognitive Behavior Therapy for Depression

Cognitive behavior therapy (CBT) is the most well-established psychotherapeutic treatment for major depression both as an adjunctive to ADs and as a stand-alone treatment (for less severe episodes). A systematic review and meta-analysis of a comparison of second-generation AD (SSRI, SNRI, and other receptor-specific ADs) treatment versus CBT for a single episode of depression concluded that there was no difference in treatment effects, either singly or in combination (Amick et al., 2015). *Cognitive therapy* (see Paykel et al., 2005), including *mindfulness-based cognitive therapy* (see Ma & Teasdale, 2004; Teasdale et al., 2000), has also been shown to prevent relapses and recurrences in recurrent major depression. A recent 2-year follow-up study of 289 individuals with recurrent major depression did not find continued AD treatment superior to preventive cognitive therapy provided while tapering AD in terms of risk of relapse and recovery (Bockting et al., 2018). *Well-being therapy*, a modification of CBT, was also shown useful in preventing relapses (see Fava, Rafanelli, Cazzaro, Conti, & Grandi, 1998).

Behavioral Activation

Behavioral activation is a well-recognized addition to treatment for depression. In a four-arm, randomized controlled study of 241 patients with major depression (mean Hamilton Depression Rating Scale [HAM-D] score was 20.74) it was found that behavioral activation and AD had equal efficacy and both were more efficacious than cognitive therapy or placebo at initial treatment (Dimidjian et al., 2006). An extension of this study examined the efficacy of the same interventions for preventing recurrences and found that both behavioral activation and cognitive therapy were as efficacious as AD (Dobson et al., 2008). Adding behavioral activation as an intervention may prove to be a key intervention in deprescribing ADs.

Exercise Training

Exercise has emerged as a close-to-equivalent treatment for depression. In a randomized controlled trial of 156 depressed individuals aged 50 or older, treatment with AD was compared to exercise or a combination of the two. All three groups showed a similarly significant drop in HAM-D scores at the end of 16 weeks (Blumenthal et al., 1999). The same participants were reevaluated at 10 months, and it was seen that the exercise group had a lower recurrence rate than the medication group (Babyak et al., 2000). A consideration with exercise is level of motivation and follow through—developing an consistent regimen is a challenge for most people without depression, and additional symptoms could present difficulties with follow through in the implementation for the person. At the same time, the side effects of this intervention cross multiple domains, making it an appealing option as a supplemental intervention.

Conclusion

In the past decade, AD medications have been mired in controversy over their effectiveness as well as more recently their potential contribution to the pathophysiology of some recurrent depressive episodes. The deprescribing of ADs requires thorough planning and preparation for management of potential withdrawal symptoms and prevention of future recurrences of depression by using slow tapers, AD switches, and psychotherapeutic interventions. Primary care physicians, who constitute the bulk of AD prescribers, must be educated about the degree of distress that withdrawal symptoms can produce. Future research focused on elucidating the long-term side effects of these medications and neurobiological basis of withdrawal syndromes could assist in the further development of deprescribing protocols.

Case Examples

Case Example 1

Joe, a 25-year-old single white man, has taken escitalopram 20 mg/d for more than 6 years following a single major depressive episode precipitated by a relationship break-up (during which he had suicidal ideation). He currently lives in his own apartment, has a part-time job, and is taking online classes. He smokes marijuana once a week but does not drink alcohol or use any other recreational drugs. He has had no depressive or anxiety symptoms for 3 years. He is asking about discontinuing escitalopram.

Guidelines of the American Psychiatric Association suggest that a patient can attempt discontinuation of the AD after 9 months of treatment if they have had only one episode of depression. In Joe's case, this guideline is applicable. The risks of ongoing escitalopram use for Joe, are mainly related to sexual dysfunction which can be very distressing for a 25-year-old man, while the continued benefits are unclear. The main risks of discontinuation are the withdrawal symptoms and a potential future recurrence that might have been prevented by escitalopram. Although his initial episode was severe, the risk of recurrence for Joe is not clearly known. Joe's consent around this risk/benefit calculation should be obtained, along with a plan for the management of withdrawal symptoms and a personalized list of symptoms and strategies to identify and manage a recurrence (see Table 8.2).

Table 8.2 Decision-making grid for case 1

Decision-making grid		
	Risks	Benefits
Continuing escitalopram	Long-term side effects including sexual dysfunction	Possible prevention of recurrence
Deprescribing escitalopram	Withdrawal symptoms Time and labor-intensive process Possible recurrence of depression	Development of non-pharmacological strategies Patient wishes to deprescribe

Patient values/preference: Patient prefers to risk a recurrence of depression rather than continue escitalopram at this point

Plan: Deprescribe escitalopram

Interventions: Psychoeducation about withdrawal symptoms, bolstering social support, lifestyle changes, CBT, cessation of marijuana, developing a relapse prevention plan

Case Example 2

Jill, a 34-year-old white woman, is on venlafaxine for management of re-current major depression. She has had three episodes in the past, the last one (a year ago) causing her to be hospitalized due to an overdose of 10 pills of aspirin. She says that she has weighed the benefits of continuing venlafaxine against the risks and side effects and feels like she does not want to take any medication for depression anymore.

Jill has had three episodes of depression, including one severe enough to cause hospitalization. Guidelines would clearly indicate that she should continue taking ADs (see Table 8.3) and this needs to be clearly communicated to Jill. This is an opportunity to engage in exploration of undisclosed side effects and the meaning of medications (and diagnosis) for Jill. Non-pharmacological strategies can be added either way to en-sure minimum effective dosing. Psychoeducation can be provided and the alliance bolstered, even if Jill accepts your recommendation not to change the regimen. Careful attention should be paid to the possibility that Jill will decide to discontinue the medications on her own, and clear messaging to Jill that rather than discontinue on her own, there is a pos-sible reduction strategy with which she can collaborate on. The risk-benefit of medication discontinuation without prescriber knowledge,

Table 8.3 Decision-making grid for case 2

Decision-making grid		
	Risks	Benefits
Continuing venlafaxine	Patient may drop out of treatment if she feels that her thoughts are being disregarded Side effects	Prevention of recurrence (she is at a high risk for recurrence as she has had three past episodes and has been suicidal in at least one)
Deprescribing venlafaxine	Withdrawal symptoms Time and labor-intensive process Recurrence of symptoms	Increased focus on other contributors to depression Patient prefers to deprescribe

Patient values/preference: Patient has strongly expressed a preference for not taking AD

Plan: Further exploration of meaning of medications and of the patient's decision-making process

Interventions: Psychoeducation about withdrawal symptoms, bolstering social support, lifestyle changes, CBT, developing a relapse prevention plan or WRAP plan

versus non adherence to guidelines and supporting a collaborative trial of medication reduction, should be thoroughly explored. If necessary, seeking peer consultation and identifying prescriber biases will be useful in decision making here.

Case Example 3

Jack, a 37-year-old man with bipolar depression and alcohol use disorder, takes lithium 1,500 mg a day (level 1.00 mEq/L) and amitriptyline 100 mg qHS, continues to drink, and has ongoing mild to moderate depressive symptoms. He says that he does not want to be on two medications.

Since Jack has bipolar disorder, the use of an AD is controversial (see the STEP-BD recommendations). Furthermore, he continues to have symptoms even though he is taking an AD (albeit at a low dose). To add to this, Jack continues to drink alcohol daily, which could be significantly exacerbating his depressive symptoms. In this situation, Jack might be advised to taper amitriptyline, start CBTi for predicted emergent insomnia, and assess Jack's stage of change around his alcohol use in order to decide on possible interventions. Distinct

Table 8.4 Decision-making grid for case 3

Decision-making grid

	Risks	Benefits
Continuing amitriptyline	Conversion to rapid cycling Anticholinergic side effects	Some improvement in depressive symptoms Management of neuropathic pain
Deprescribing amitriptyline	Withdrawal symptoms Time and labor-intensive process Increase in depressive symptoms	Increased focus on other contributors to depression including alcohol use Patient prefers to deprescribe

Patient values/preference: Patient prefers to take only one medication

Plan: Deprescribe amitriptyline

Interventions: Psychoeducation about withdrawal symptoms, bolstering social support, lifestyle changes, CBT, cessation of alcohol use, developing relapse prevention or WRAP plan

from serotonergic effects, he may experience symptoms of cholinergic rebound that could be managed by either slowing the taper of the primary medication or adding a pure anticholinergic agent (such as benztropine) for a short taper (see Table 8.4). In addition, doing a thorough assessment of Jack's current life situation and looking at contributing contextual factors will inform recommendation of other possible adjunctive supports.

Case Example 4

Anna, a 78-year-old woman who lives with her family, ambulates on a scooter due to osteoarthritis, has chronic obstructive pulmonary disease, and is taking multiple medications. She was given mirtazapine 30mg QHS 7 years ago, which was augmented with bupropion 150 mg 3 years ago, and she has continued the combination since then.

There are no guidelines for the duration of treatment with an AD that has been added to augment an initial. In this case, the prescriber might initiate a discussion recommending the deprescribing of bupropion to minimize drug interactions and side effects (see Table 8.5).

Table 8.5 Decision-making grid for case 5

Decision-making grid		
	Risks	Benefits
Continuing bupropion	Long-term side effects including lowering of seizure threshold and increased blood pressure Drug interactions	No evidence for benefits of continuation
Deprescribing bupropion	Withdrawal symptoms Increase in depressive symptoms	Reduced side effect Reduced risk of interactions leading to adverse outcomes

Patient values/preference: Patient prefers fewer medications but leaves the decision up to you

Plan: Deprescribe bupropion

Interventions: Psychoeducation about withdrawal symptoms, monitor for recurrence

Self-Assessment

1. **Joan is a 56-year-old married woman who has taken duloxetine 60 mg twice a day for more than 6 years. Before she started taking duloxetine, she had three episodes of mild to moderate depression in a span of 5 years. She has never been actively suicidal or hospitalized and is otherwise healthy. She is asking about the possibility of discontinuing duloxetine.**
   a. What are you most inclined to recommend?
   b. If Joan asks for more information, what are the factors you will consider and advise her on?
   c. If Joan decides that she wants to discontinue duloxetine, what are the withdrawal symptoms you will warn her about?

2. **Tim is a 30-year-old single man who experienced a severe episode of depression 3 years ago following the death of his best friend. He was neither experiencing psychosis nor hospitalized, but he had suicidal**

ideation. He has been taking citalopram 20 mg and is doing well. Would you suggest tapering off citalopram?

a. What would you recommend and why?

b. What will you do if Tim refuses to taper off citalopram despite your suggestion?

c. What will you do if Tim insists on stopping the medication despite your suggestion?

3. Karen is a 40-year-old woman who continued to have depressive symptoms despite taking sertraline 200 mg for over 12 weeks. You give her bupropion 300 mg as augmentation, and the symptoms subside over the next 6 weeks. She is now asking about how long she needs to take the medications.

a. Would you recommend continuing both medications? Justify your recommendation.

b. If you recommend tapering, which medication would you recommend and why?

Recommended Reading

Amick, H. R., Gartlehner, G., Gaynes, B. N., Forneris, C., Asher, G. N., Morgan, L. C., . . . Gaylord, S. (2015). Comparative benefits and harms of second generation antidepressants and cognitive behavioral therapies in initial treatment of major depressive disorder: systematic review and meta-analysis. *British Medical Journal, 351*, h6019.

Babyak, M., Blumenthal, J. A., Herman, S., Khatri, P., Doraiswamy, M., Moore, K., . . . Krishnan, K. R. (2000). Exercise treatment for major depression: maintenance of therapeutic benefit at 10 months. *Psychosomatic Medicine, 62*(5), 633–638.

Baumeister, H. (2012). Inappropriate prescriptions of antidepressant drugs in patients with subthreshold to mild depression: Time for the evidence to become practice. *Journal of Affective Disorders, 139*(3), 240–243.

Berwian, I. M., Walter, H., Seifritz, E., & Huys, Q. J. (2017). Predicting relapse after antidepressant withdrawal–a systematic review. *Psychological Medicine, 47*(3), 426–437.

Blumenthal, J. A., Babyak, M. A., Moore, K. A., Craighead, W. E., Herman, S., Khatri, P., . . . Appelbaum, M. (1999). Effects of exercise training on older patients with major depression. *Archives of Internal Medicine*, *159*(19), 2349–2356.

Bockting, C. L., Klein, N. S., Elgersma, H. J., van Rijsbergen, G. D., Slofstra, C., Ormel, J., . . . Nolen, W. A. (2018). Effectiveness of preventive cognitive therapy while tapering antidepressants versus maintenance antidepressant treatment versus their combination in prevention of depressive relapse or recurrence (DRD study): A three-group, multicentre, randomised controlled trial. *The Lancet Psychiatry*, *5*(5), 401–410.

Byrne, S. E., & Rothschild, A. J. (1998). Loss of antidepressant efficacy during maintenance therapy: possible mechanisms and treatments. *The Journal of Clinical Psychiatry*, *59*(6), 279–288.

Chouinard, G., & Chouinard, V.-A. (2015). New classification of selective serotonin reuptake inhibitor withdrawal. *Psychotherapy and Psychosomatics*, *84*(2), 63–71.

Clarke, K., Mayo-Wilson, E., Kenny, J., & Pilling, S. (2015). Can non-pharmacological interventions prevent relapse in adults who have recovered from depression? A systematic review and meta-analysis of randomised controlled trials. *Clinical Psychology Review*, *39*, 58–70.

Cosci, F. (2017). Withdrawal symptoms after discontinuation of a noradrenergic and specific serotonergic antidepressant: A case report and review of the literature. *Personalized Medicine in Psychiatry*, *1*, 81–84.

Dilsaver, S. C., Feinberg, M., & Greden, J. F. (1983). Antidepressant withdrawal symptoms treated with anticholinergic agents. *American Journal of Psychiatry*, *140*(2), 249–251.

Dimidjian, S., Hollon, S. D., Dobson, K. S., Schmaling, K. B., Kohlenberg, R. J., Addis, M. E., . . . Gollan, J. K. (2006). Randomized trial of behavioral activation, cognitive therapy, and antidepressant medication in the acute treatment of adults with major depression. *Journal of Consulting and Clinical Psychology*, *74*(4), 658.

Dobson, K. S., Hollon, S. D., Dimidjian, S., Schmaling, K. B., Kohlenberg, R. J., Gallop, R. J., . . . Jacobson, N. S. (2008). Randomized trial of behavioral activation, cognitive therapy, and antidepressant medication in the prevention of relapse and recurrence in major depression. *Journal of Consulting and Clinical Psychology*, *76*(3), 468.

El-Mallakh, R. S., Gao, Y., & Roberts, R. J. (2011). Tardive dysphoria: the role of long term antidepressant use in-inducing chronic depression. *Medical Hypotheses*, *76*(6), 769–773.

Eveleigh, R., Muskens, E., Lucassen, P., Verhaak, P., Spijker, J., van Weel, C., . . . Speckens, A. (2017). Withdrawal of unnecessary antidepressant medication: a randomised controlled trial in primary care. *BJGP Open, 1*(4), BJGP-2017-0169. doi: 10.3399/bjgpopen17X101265

Fava, G. A. (2018). Time to rethink the approach to recurrent depression. *The Lancet Psychiatry, 5*(5), 380–381.

Fava, G. A., Rafanelli, C., Cazzaro, M., Conti, S., & Grandi, S. (1998). Well-being therapy. A novel psychotherapeutic approach for residual symptoms of affective disorders. *Psychological Medicine, 28*(2), 475–480.

Fava, M. (2000). Weight gain and antidepressants. *The Journal of Clinical Psychiatry, 61,* 37–41.

Frank, E., Prien, R., Jarrett, R., Keller, M., Kupfer, D., Lavori, P., . . . Weissman, M. (1991). Conceptualization and rationale for consensus definitions of terms in major depressive disorder. *Archives of General Psychiatry, 48*(9), 851–855.

Geddes, J. R., Carney, S. M., Davies, C., Furukawa, T. A., Kupfer, D. J., Frank, E., & Goodwin, G. M. (2003). Relapse prevention with antidepressant drug treatment in depressive disorders: A systematic review. *The Lancet, 361*(9358), 653–661.

Groot, P. C., & van Os, J. (2018). Antidepressant tapering strips to help people come off medication more safely. *Psychosis,* 1–4.

Haddad, P. M. (2001). Antidepressant discontinuation syndromes. *Drug Safety, 24*(3), 183–197.

Keller, M. B., & Boland, R. J. (1998). Implications of failing to achieve successful long-term maintenance treatment of recurrent unipolar major depression. *Biological Psychiatry, 44*(5), 348–360.

Lejoyeux, M., & Adès, J. (1997). Antidepressant discontinuation: A review of the literature. *The Journal of Clinical Psychiatry, 58*(Suppl 7), 11–16.

Lejoyeux, M., Adès, J., Mourad, S., Solomon, J., & Dilsaver, S. (1996). Antidepressant withdrawal syndrome. *CNS Drugs, 5*(4), 278–292.

Li, Y., Pehrson, A. L., Budac, D. P., Sánchez, C., & Gulinello, M. (2012). A rodent model of premenstrual dysphoria: progesterone withdrawal induces depression-like behavior that is differentially sensitive to classes of antidepressants. *Behavioural brain research, 234*(2), 238–247.

Ma, S. H., & Teasdale, J. D. (2004). Mindfulness-based cognitive therapy for depression: Replication and exploration of differential relapse prevention effects. *Journal of Consulting and Clinical Psychology, 72*(1), 31.

Nierenberg, A. A., Petersen, T. J., & Alpert, J. E. (2003). Prevention of relapse and recurrence in depression: The role of long-term pharmacotherapy and psychotherapy. *Journal of Clinical Psychiatry, 64*(15), 13–17.

Paykel, E., Scott, J., Cornwall, P., Abbott, R., Crane, C., Pope, M., & Johnson, A. (2005). Duration of relapse prevention after cognitive therapy in residual depression: Follow-up of controlled trial. *Psychological Medicine, 35*(1), 59–68.

Perahia, D. G., Kajdasz, D. K., Desaiah, D., & Haddad, P. M. (2005). Symptoms following abrupt discontinuation of duloxetine treatment in patients with major depressive disorder. *Journal of Affective Disorders, 89*(1), 207–212.

Prien, R. F., & Kupfer, D. J. (1986). Continuation drug therapy for major depressive episodes: How long should it be maintained? *American Journal of Psychiatry, 143*(1), 18–23.

Reeves, R. R., Mack, J. E., & Beddingfield, J. J. (2003). Shock-like sensations during venlafaxine withdrawal. *Pharmacotherapy: The Journal of Human Pharmacology and Drug Therapy, 23*(5), 678–681.

Teasdale, J. D., Segal, Z. V., Williams, J. M. G., Ridgeway, V. A., Soulsby, J. M., & Lau, M. A. (2000). Prevention of relapse/recurrence in major depression by mindfulness-based cognitive therapy. *Journal of Consulting and Clinical Psychology, 68*(4), 615.

Therrien, F., & Markowitz, J. S. (1997). Selective serotonin reuptake inhibitors and withdrawal symptoms: A review of the literature. *Human Psychopharmacology: Clinical and Experimental, 12*(4), 309–323.

Warner, C. H., Bobo, W., Warner, C., Reid, S., & Rachal, J. (2006). Antidepressant discontinuation syndrome. *American Family Physician, 74*(3), 449–456.

9

Deprescribing Antipsychotic Medications

In this chapter, we present specific context, considerations and clinical decision-making relevant to deprescribing antipsychotics. We apply the same caveats found in the introduction to chapter 8 and urge the reader to consider this work through their own critical lens of knowledge, experience and expertise. A specific challenge for this class of medications is the broad receptor profiles, growing set of clinical indications, considerable off-label use and diagnostic uncertainty that dispels all but the most robust fantasies of therapeutic precision. The principal focus of deprescribing in this chapter may well be the pursuit of minimum effective dosing more than complete discontinuation, excepting the case of multiple antipsychotic medications. Issues of shared decision making and informed consent are particularly pertinent when working with vulnerable populations such as those experiencing psychotic disorders. We discuss here factors that might recommend for and against deprescribing antipsychotic medications (APs). We also describe the clinical presentation and management of related rebound and discontinuation syndromes. Finally, we integrate some nonpharmacological interventions that may support deprescribing these medications when indicated.

Goals and Learning Objectives

After reading this chapter, the reader will be able to:

1. Frame a risk benefit calculation for ongoing prescriptions of APs for a given clinical scenario
2. List common symptoms of AP and anticholinergic discontinuation syndromes and their management
3. Develop an AP deprescribing plan for a given patient

Case Example

Graham is a 49-year-old white man who lives with his elderly mother in a third-floor walk-up apartment. He has been diagnosed with treatment refractory schizophrenia, and his chart indicates he was prescribed five different antipsychotic medications (with an unclear adequacy of trials) before being initiated on clozapine 1 year ago in addition to continuing haloperidol 10mg at bedtime which he states helps with sleep. Although the combination of clozapine and haloperidol provided him the best response in terms of further reducing his subjective distress around auditory hallucinations, these experiences continue on a daily basis, and he has learned to cope with them to a degree. Graham has gained more than 100 pounds since starting clozapine and has developed type 2 diabetes, heart disease, and osteoarthritis in his knees, limiting his ability to leave home.

The discontinuation of APs is one of the more contentious issues in psychiatric deprescribing (see Table 9.1 for common AP medications and their indications). The level of uncertainty that surrounds the etiology and heterogeneity of the condition(s) of schizophrenia spectrum disorders, the often chaotic and functionally impactful presentations of illness, the prevalent stigma and misconceptions that surround them, the increasingly burdensome long-term side-effect profiles (notable metabolic side effects of atypical APs), the cost of care and related disability, and lack of cohesiveness and clarity in the research literature, among countless other factors, confound the best-intentioned prescriber embarking on a shared decision-making process.

Deprescribing offers a framework for the periodic reassessment of medication risk–benefit ratios and for their optimal, collaborative reduction to the minimum effective dose and discontinuation when indicated. Current guidelines for the treatment of patients with schizophrenia and other chronic psychotic disorders state that APs are critical to controlling symptoms of psychosis *and preventing relapse* (emphasis added, APA, 2006). The evidence base for APs is strongest in favor of treatment of acute agitation (hence APs are also known as "major tranquilizers") and positive symptoms (such as auditory hallucinations), but unfortunately less so for addressing the negative and cognitive symptoms which more closely predict

Table 9.1 Commonly prescribed antipsychotic medications

Class	Common medications	Common uses
Atypical antipsychotics	Risperidone, paliperidone, olanzapine, quetiapine, clozapine, ziprasidone, aripiprazole	Schizophrenia (and some: bipolar disorder and unipolar depression) Some: acute agitation, behavioral disturbances associated with dementia, Parkinson's disease, behavioral dysregulation in children and adolescents, problems with impulse control
Typical antipsychotics	Haloperidol, fluphenazine, perphenazine, chlorpromazine	Psychotic disorders H: Tourette's, second-line for severe behavioral problems in children C: nausea/vomiting, acute intermittent porphyria, mania, tetanus, intractable hiccups, combativeness in children. Bipolar disorder, acute agitation
Anticholinergics	Benztropine, trihexyphenidyl	Parkinson's disease, extrapyramidal symptoms (related to antipsychotic use)

functional impact. The prevailing evidence demands APs be started and specialized care be sought as quickly as possible after psychotic symptoms emerge with the goal of reducing duration of untreated psychosis, associated with worse prognosis. When schizophrenia is (often later) diagnosed, large retrospective epidemiological studies support the notion that APs need to be continued indefinitely at the minimum effective dose to prevent relapse of this commonly relapsing and remitting condition. However, diagnostic uncertainty can persist, with those who may not need continuous maintenance treatment difficult to identify. Consider for example Ian, a 21 year old man who remains well 1 year following his initial, and only, 2 month episode of psychosis with some features of mania and coincident cannabis use and faithfully continues maintenance treatment with an AP. He reports some decreased motivation and difficulty concentrating preventing him from returning to college. His affect is constricted. Does Ian suffer from schizophrenia? Could this have been a prolonged cannabis-induced psychosis? Could this be a primary bipolar I disorder? Could his apparent negative and cognitive symptoms be purely side effects of the AP? We may not have a definitive answer until the AP is withdrawn—but at what risk?

Although the field has characterized and coalesced around a prevailing model for psychosis and its treatment (i.e. mesolimbic hyperdopaminergia driving aberrant salience, tempered by D2 receptor antagonism), exceptions such as the relatively low D2 receptor affinity of our most effective AP, clozapine, and the burgeoning glutamatergic model of psychosis, muddy the waters. Uncertainty further abounds when considering that a recommendation to continue APs indefinitely is typically predicated on a phenomenological diagnosis of schizophrenia—currently best understood as a syndrome without a universally accepted pathoetiology or diagnostic test. Indeed, psychosis as a symptom can occur in a range of conditions with vastly varying etiologies and prognoses. For example, a substance-induced psychotic episode may remit spontaneously within a week or so with cessation of the substance. Newer clinical guidelines speak to continuing APs for at least 6 months to a year after a first episode of psychosis before reviewing; however, the largely longterm, retrospective, observational studies generally showing discontinuation after 1 year as being detrimental are limited by potential confounds such as illness severity, changing environmental factors (such as potency of cannabis), limited inference of causality and lack of agreement on most meaningful patient-centered outcomes. We further cannot yet confidently predict those individuals who will benefit from continued prescription and those who would benefit from deprescribing. These reflections are not intended to undermine the value of our diagnostic classifications, nor the research methods currently at our disposal which have been put to good use providing illuminating clinical research and new treatments providing life-altering benefits. However, we do intend to highlight the need for further work in this area, as well as our responsibility to acknowledge and address the uncertainty and imprecision that remains at this time inherent in the holistic management of any individual presenting with psychotic experiences.

Specific guidelines for treatment of schizophrenia show more concordance in the acute than in the maintenance phase of treatment. This might reflects, in part, the relative glut of short-term efficacy trials over long-term effectiveness data. The American Psychiatric Association (APA, 2006) and the World Federation of Societies of Biological Psychiatry (Hasan et al., 2012) recommend continuing the same regimen to which the patient has responded for at least 6 months, and the International Psychopharmacology Algorithm Project (Takeuchi, Suzuki, Uchida, Watanabe, & Mimura, 2012;) recommends maintaining the dose that was effective in the acute phase during the first few months. Maintenance dosing guidelines recommend chlorpromazine equivalents of 600 mg/d or less (see Hasan et al.,

2012; Kreyenbuhl, Buchanan, Dickerson, & Dixon, 2010) or haloperidol equivalents of 8 mg/d or less (roughly equivalent to a chlorpromazine-equivalent dose of 400 mg).

Potential Consequences of Long-Term
AP pharmacotherapy

AP Polypharmacy

Rates of AP polypharmacy have risen over the past two decades (see Essock, Covell et al., 2009; Ganguly, Kotzan et al., 2004)—arguably ahead of the evidence supporting potential benefits (i.e. in treatment refractory cases) over the risk of additive side effects. There are other examples in medicine, where clinical practice has led the clinical research, though the approach has benefits and drawbacks. Although the literature supporting rational AP polypharmacy does continue to grow, the evidence remains circumscribed. Due to lack of guidelines for AP polypharmacy, AP combinations are at risk of being continued indefinitely (see Stahl & Grady, 2004). Encouragingly for example, some studies have shown that a large proportion of patients can be safely transitioned from multiple APs to a single AP without incident (e.g. Borlido, Remington et al., 2016), although others report worse outcomes (e.g. Katona, Czobor et al., 2014). At this point in time, with limited evidence for the use of multiple APs for extended periods it is incumbent to carefully consider the risks as they apply to each individual patient.

Risk–Benefit Ratios Shift with Increasing Age and
Duration of Illness

The margin of error in our risk–benefit calculation increases with duration of treatment largely due to a lack of longer-term effectiveness studies. Without clearly reliable predictors of relapse, deprescribing guidelines, and tenable alternatives, well-intentioned prescribers may be biased towards recommending longer courses and higher than necessary doses than may be necessary. From a public health perspective, the conservative position, risking 'over-treating' may be defended if it were not for the crisis of increased metabolic syndrome and cardiovascular mortality in this population linked to continued atypical AP use.

Murray (2016) proposes the controversial hypothesis that treatment with APs may compound the primary hyperdopaminergic state in psychosis by producing a secondary *dopamine supersensitivity*. This mechanism has been propose to explain the construct of withdrawal/rebound psychosis (upon abrupt AP discontinuation) which some authors argue is a potential iatrogenic concern requiring attention (see Moncrieff, 2006). Although some experts conclude that there is insufficient evidence of significant neurological sequelae (see Goff, 2017), the metabolic and cardiovascular consequences are indisputable (see Saha et al., 2007). As age and medical comorbidities increase, the risks of indefinitely continuing APs unchanged may begin to outweigh projected benefits, a concept well-addressed in geriatric medication (see the Beer's Criteria). Age-related changes in pharmacokinetics and dynamics warrant the periodic review of medications and predict the need for the reduction of particular agents, such as anticholinergics and sedatives which can lead to cognitive impairment and increased falls, respectively. Some APs, with their broad receptor profiles (notably those with significant anticholinergic and antihistaminergic) as well as central nervous system depressant effects, should be routinely considered for deprescribing (dose reduction, switch, or discontinuation) with advancing age. The possibility of remission of psychotic illness as patients age may also be considered and emphasizes the importance of reviewing AP dosage and necessity on a regular basis.

Factors Contributing to the Extended Use of Antipsychotic Medications

The argument for deprescribing APs is more easily made when there is diagnostic uncertainty or a high likelihood that the recent psychotic episode may have been a one-time event or secondary to a medical cause, primary mood disorder or substance use. Schizophrenia, however, when apparent, is understood to commonly take a life-long relapsing and remitting course that is amenable to management but not cure. A key decision point, one potentially determining a patient's longer term care, comes after remission of a first episode of psychosis. A common belief is that life-long treatment with APs is needed and, indeed, there is little evidence to support safe AP discontinuation after the first year of treatment (see Tihonen et al., 2018). Several studies have demonstrated high rates of relapse following AP reduction (Chen, Hui et al., 2010; Zipursky et al., 2014). Overall, the efficacy of APs for the initial treatment of psychosis is well established, but more research is needed to determine whether some individuals may respond to alternative pharmacologic or nonpharmacologic treatments and, if so, how to identify which treatments and for which patients (Goff, Falkai et al., 2017). While this is a controversial area and a topic that arouses strong sentiment on either side of the debate, the stance of embracing the possibility that each patient's individual circumstances, course of illness, preferences, and changing life circumstances may not fall in line with guidelines and deserves consideration is in line with person-centered approaches.

Overall, studies show that discontinuation is associated with relapse in a significantly higher proportion of patients diagnosed with chronic psychotic disorders than in those who continue medications (Gilbert, Harris et al., 1995; Leucht, Tardy et al., 2012; Viguera, Baldessarini et al., 1997; Zipursky, Menezes et al., 2014). However, these studies, other than having varying definitions of relapse, have particular inferential limitations for deprescribing. Many do not individualize the medication taper, and in some cases, stop the medications abruptly. Adjunctive psychosocial offerings are not a formal part of protocols in these trials, differentiating them from a deprescribing effort as put forth here. To reiterate, AP *discontinuation* is not equivalent to AP *deprescribing*.

The majority of AP discontinuation studies conclude that there is a subset of patients who may not require indefinite AP treatment, and, although commonly understood, guidelines do not yet exist to support practice for that subset. For example, one study reports that 40% of patients whose symptoms remit after a first episode may have a good outcome with either no or minimal AP treatment (Murray, Quattrone et al., 2016). An individualized risk calculator for predicting successful deprescribing of APs would be hugely valuable to the field—one such tool has been developed to predict conversion to full psychosis in those with clinical high risk syndrome (Cannon et al., 2016). A similar methodology could be employed here.

As noted in Table 9.1, the range of clinical indications for APs stretch beyond the treatment of schizophrenia and continue to expand. Atypical APs are becoming first line for the acute, and even maintenance, treatment of bipolar disorder and the treatment of bipolar as well as unipolar (adjunctive) depression. Independent of an affective or psychotic disorder, APs are now widely prescribed for acute agitation and behavioral problems in children and people with dementia (Findling, Steiner et al., 2004; Park, Cervesi et al., 2016). The use of quetiapine for insomnia (Coe & Hong, 2012; Anderson, Vande, & Griend, 2014) and atypical APs for posttraumatic stress disorder (Hermes, Sernyak et al., 2014) has become more prevalent and provide further examples of real-world clinical practice advancing, for better or for worse, ahead of research evidence. Again, with limited published guidance around AP use for these burgeoning indications, discontinuation may be disincentivized. Whether the apparent versatility of atypical AP justifies their broadening use remains to be proved empirically.

Another factor potentially driving indefinite use of APs is that management of schizophrenia has largely focused on remission of *symptoms* rather than on functional *recovery*. This questions whether we are targeting meaningful, achievable, and person-centered outcomes with our treatments versus strictly symptom control. Definitions of remission refer to improvement in the core symptoms of psychosis such that they no longer interfere with behavior (and are at a threshold lower than the one used for the initial diagnosis of schizophrenia—e.g., on a rating scale such as the Positive and Negative Syndrome Scale [PANSS]; Andreasen, Carpenter Jr. et al., 2005). Recovery, in contrast, is a fuller concept, reflecting a person's ability to lead a meaningful and fulfilled life and maximizing (1) autonomy based on that patient's desires and capabilities, (2) dignity and self-respect, (3) participation and integration into full community life, and (4) resumption of normal development. The concept of recovery has been highly endorsed by the APA (2005) as well as by the US federal government (New Freedom Commission on Mental Health, 2003). Functional recovery takes time and may therefore pose a less attractive outcome measure for clinical trials with follow-up durations limited by feasibility and cost.

Thomas Insel, former Director of the National Institute of Mental Health (NIMH), reflected that "although these symptoms [of psychosis] can be frightening and dangerous for patients, family members, and providers, APs safely and effectively help people through the crisis of acute psychosis. However, the long-term management of chronic mental illness is another matter. Recently, results from several studies have suggested that these medications may be less effective for the outcomes that matter most to people with serious mental illness: a full return to well-being and a productive place in society."

Focusing on a broader measure of *recovery* (encapsulating symptomatic and functional outcomes), Wunderink et al. (2007) conducted a clinical trial in people in 6-month remission with APs following a first episode of psychosis, randomized to maintenance treatment with APs or *guided* dose reduction or discontinuation. Over the initial 18-month follow-up period the relapse rate in the dose reduction group was twice that of the maintenance group; however, at 7 years, those persons in the dose reduction arm showed greater functional recovery and comparable symptomatic recovery as compared to medication maintenance (see Wunderink, Nieboer et al., 2013). Furthermore, the Chicago follow-up study for example, which tracked individuals for 20 years after a first episode of psychosis, reported that those not on APs had better *functional* outcomes than those who continued APs (Harrow & Jobe, 2013). Table 9.2 summarizes studies looking at relapse rates following AP discontinuation.

Discontinuation Syndromes

A special consideration when deprescribing APs is the reappearance of psychotic symptoms during the process. This reappearance of symptoms can be understood as a rebound of the underlying illness but has alternatively been hypothesized to represent a 'supersensitivity' or 'withdrawal psychosis' by some. *Supersensitivity psychosis* has been defined as the appearance of new psychotic symptoms (or psychotic symptoms of greater severity) in a patient who abruptly discontinues or reduces APs after chronic use (see Chouinard, 1991). However, this concept does not have broad acceptance, and its mechanism has not been elucidated (Goff, 2015). Another reported withdrawal syndrome attributable to dopaminergic function is withdrawal-emergent dyskinesia (a subtype of TD) which typically resolves spontaneously over 1–2 months after abrupt AP cessation. Reintroduction of the AP and gradual taper over several months can help.

Abrupt discontinuation of an AP with high anticholinergic effects (such as clozapine) as well as the anticholinergic agents commonly used as adjuncts to AP treatment may precipitate a cholinergic rebound involving nausea, malaise, diaphoresis, and tachycardia. Although no specific guidelines exist,

Table 9.2 Summary of systematic reviews examining relapse rates following antipsychotic (AP) discontinuation in schizophrenia

	Reference	Methodology	Findings	Conclusions	Limitations
1.	Gilbert, Harris et al., 1995	Systematic review of 66 studies of AP withdrawal in schizophrenia	Over a mean follow-up period of 9.7 months the relapse rate was 53% in patients who discontinued AP and 17% in those who did not.	Risk–benefit of neuroleptic continuation Vs taper must be considered carefully.	AP withdrawn in 1 day in 42 studies, 24 studies had a taper duration between 2 and 60 days 22 studies did not provide a definition of relapse No mention of psychosocial interventions
2.	Viguera, Baldessarini et al., 1997	Systematic review of AP discontinuation in studies 1,210 patients with schizophrenia	After abrupt discontinuation, the risk of relapse reached 50% within 6 months.	The risk of relapse was highest within 6 months of discontinuing AP. Subjects who remained stable in the first 6 months were more likely to remain stable after	In 1,006 of the 1,210 patients, AP was discontinued abruptly No mention of psychosocial interventions
3.	Chen, Hui et al., 2010	178 patients with first episode psychosis maintained on quetiapine vs. placebo for 1 year	Relapse at 12 months was 41% (95% confidence interval, 29–53%) for the quetiapine group and 79% (68–90%) for the placebo group	Quetiapine treatment substantially reduced the risk of relapse in first episode psychosis patients	No mention of psychosocial factors or treatments

No.	Study	Method	Results	Conclusion	Limitations
4.	Leucht, Tardy et al., 2012	Meta-analysis of 65 trials involving 6,500 patients	APs significantly reduced relapse rates at 1 year (drugs 27% vs. placebo 64%). Fewer patients given APs than placebo were readmitted (10% vs. 26%) but less than a third of relapsed patients had to be admitted. In a meta-regression, the difference between drug and placebo decreased with study length.	APs benefit patients with schizophrenia. More data needs to be obtained about the long-term morbidity and mortality of APs.	The funnel plot was asymmetrical and may represent a small trial effect Time to relapse data was not available for most studies Method of PA withdrawal was not described No mention of psychosocial interventions
5.	Zipursky, Menezes et al., 2014	Systematic review of six studies of AP discontinuation in first-episode psychosis patients, after they had achieved symptomatic remission	Recurrence rates in the AP discontinuation group were 77% and 90% at the end of 1 and 2 years. Recurrence rates in the AP continuation group were 3%.	Trial off AP medications in first-episode psychosis patients is not recommended as the risk of recurrence is very high	Three studies discontinued AP over a maximum of 3 months, two studies stopped depot AP, one did not specify the rate of discontinuation Variable definitions of recurrence

Table 9.3 Discontinuation syndromes related to antipsychotic prescription and suggested management

Symptom	Mechanism	Management
Nausea, malaise, diaphoresis, vomiting, insomnia (Lacoursiere, Spohn et al., 1976; Cerovecki, Musil et al., 2013)	Cholinergic rebound	No specific treatment may be needed, continue anticholinergic medication for a week after discontinuing AP
Withdrawal emergent dyskinesia (Dufresne & Wagner, 1988; Chouinard 1991; Chouinard & Chouinard, 2008)	Dopamine supersensitivity	Lower the rate of taper
Decreased REM latency, REM sleep and total sleep time (Thaker, Wagman et al., 1989)	Dopamine supersensitivity	Other measures for management of insomnia such as low dose benzodiazepines, antihistaminics or trazodone
Withdrawal akathisia (Dufresne & Wagner, 1988)	Dopamine supersensitivity	Slow the rate of taper

pure anticholinergic agents may be (re)introduced and more slowly tapered. See Table 9.3 for a summary of some discontinuation syndromes related to stopping AP medications and suggested management of them.

Strategies to Support AP Deprescribing

When attempting to deprescribe an AP, consider using the seven steps outlined in Chapter 7 while paying particular attention to (1) person-centered care and outcomes, (2) shared decision-making and informed consent, (3) family involvement and other psychosocial interventions in psychosis, and (4) interactions with physical health and wellness. Again, the more common goal of a deprescribing intervention may be ensuring a minimum effective regimen rather than complete cessation of pharmacotherapy. As with other conditions and medications, the patient and their immediate circle of support are critical to the success of deprescribing through early identification of symptoms and establishing a range of nonpharmacologic coping strategies to mitigate the risk of relapse. However, due to the social aspects of chronic psychotic disorders like schizophrenia, baseline social functioning and resources may be more limited and further bolstering required.

Although the reemergence of positive psychotic symptoms may constitute an emergency for some patients, others may be quite willing and able to accept and cope with such an emergence as long as functional gains are maintained. A patient with schizophrenia, within the shared decision-making model and given adequate informed consent, should be allowed to embark upon an intervention that carries an increased risk of symptoms, distress and possibly hospitalization. The issues of capacity around such decisions may be more pertinent in psychotic disorders where symptoms such as psychotic ambivalence and reality distortion can, at times and for some, impact the decision-making process. The use of psychiatric advanced directives, more longitudinal assessment and decision-making processes, and the involvement of trusted supports and surrogate decision-makers may help. For prescribers, the ethical consideration here may warrant peer consultation and a second opinion. A particularly useful tool when deprescribing in serious mental illnesses is a Wellness Recovery Action Plan (WRAP; Copeland, 1997) which assists a person in identifying daily wellness strategies as well as early warning signs of relapse and crisis planning. WRAP empowers a person to self-monitor and intervene or seek help early if possible—however, it is noted that a "hypervigilance" to such signs of relapse can emerge.

Specific interventions might be employed to target factors such as substance use (e.g., cannabis), environmental stress, and expressed emotion that predict relapse. Cooccuring substance use is one of the strongest predictors of relapse in chronic psychotic disorders (Swofford, Kasckow et al., 1996) and its treatment is critical for relapse prevention in schizophrenia. Naltrexone or disulfiram (Petrakis, Nich et al., 2006; Petrakis et al., 2006) and motivation interviewing, cognitive behavior therapy (CBT), or family interventions (Barrowclough, Haddock et al., 2001; Drake, O'Neal et al., 2008; Barrowclough et al., 2001; Drake et al., 2008) have some evidence base. Psychotherapy such as CBT can ameliorate early symptoms accompanying a relapse such as insomnia. anxiety, or depression. As for features of psychosis itself, although a range of adjunctive psychosocial strategies have varied degrees of evidence (e.g. CBPp), none can be considered as standalone treatments or adequate replacement for a multi-faceted care plan including APs. Falloon (1982; Falloon, Boyd et al., 1982) showed that family therapy provided some addition benefit at preventing relapse over a period of months. Similarly, Hogarty (1991) demonstrated that both family psychoeducation and individual social skills training helped reduce relapse over medications alone. The effect of family psychoeducation persisted for 2 years.

Open Dialogue (a progressive approach to crisis intervention and initial care of young people experiencing psychosis) engages the individual, family, and other key supports in open discussions about all aspects of the clinical situation and decision-making. Although the evidence base remains extremely limited, this approach has been reported to provide good clinical outcomes, reduced medication utilization, and higher satisfaction with care (Gordon, Gidugu et al., 2016) and warrants further study. Table 9.4 summarizes psycho-social adjunctive interventions with some degree of evidence of benefit in schizophrenia. None of these interventions has been tested against APs in head-to-head clinical trials, and each has been trialed only in patients who were already stabilized with medications. While we suggest using these interventions to support a process of deprescribing, they cannot replace and may infact require to concomittent use of APs for optimal effects.

There are limited, conflicting guidelines for AP discontinuation. A review of studies comparing the rates of relapse with a slow versus rapid medication taper reported benefits for slow tapers (Viguera, Baldessarini et al., 1997). However, this finding was not replicated by a more recent systematic review and meta-analysis that concluded no difference in relapse rates between slow versus rapid tapers (Takeuchi, Kantor et al., 2017). A significant methodological limitation of these studies, potentially addressable by

Table 9.4 Nonpharmacological Interventions with potential benefit as adjuncts to APs for functional outcomes in schizophrenia

Type of intervention	Level of evidence	Reference
Cognitive behavior therapy	Meta-analysis	(Pilling, Bebbington et al., 2002)
Family therapy	Meta-analysis	(Pilling, Bebbington et al., 2002)
Cognitive remediation	Controlled trials	(McGurk, Twamley et al., 2007)
Psychoeducation	Meta-analysis	(McFarlane, Dixon et al., 2003)
Open dialogue	Narrative reports	(Seikkula 2001)
Hearing voices networks	Narrative reports	(Corstens, Longden et al., 2014)

future effectiveness studies of deprescribing, was that AP tapers were not individualized. Although, schedules may vary (being shorter or longer in response to specific patient and contextual factors) a reasonable starting point for duration of AP taper is 6 months. Canadian colleagues in primary care have published recommendations to deprescribe APs after 3 months when used for behavioral and psychological symptoms of dementia (this indication carries a "black box" warning in the United States) and for insomnia after any duration (Bjerre et al., 2018). This is accompanied by some guidelines for how to deprescribe APs in this context (among other resources; publicly available at *deprescribing.org* at time of writing). These authors suggest a 25–50% dose reduction every 1–2 weeks for the former indication and immediate discontinuation for insomnia. A distinction is carefully and very appropriately made, however, that these guidelines are not intended for AP deprescribing in the treatment of psychotic disorders. The methodology these authors employed to create the guideline may be useful as this field advances (see Bjerre et al., 2018).

Conclusion

Psychotic disorders, despite some diagnostic uncertainty early in their course, emerge as schizophrenia in approximately 1% of the world's population and cause profound subjective distress and chronic deleterious effects on function, with wide-ranging and significant impact on public health. Given such high stakes surrounding treatment decisions involving psychotic disorders, the question of deprescribing is contentious, and we look with urgency to a clinical literature that cannot yet provide clear guidance. Despite some more robust pockets of evidence and lines of inquiry, there remains overall uncertainty around the optimal management of psychotic disorders and the parsing out of encompassed syndromes. The clinical literature is notably limited in guiding recommendations for the duration of AP use and the proactive identification of individuals who might benefit from deprescribing. Caution should be used when attempting to generalize findings from more heterogenous first-episode psychosis cohorts to more chronic groups and vice versa. Similarly, the results of large retrospective, observational studies should be considered within the inferential limitations (of cause vs. association) inherent in their methodology. Some of these knowledge gaps may be addressed by increased interest in, and funding of, research on AP deprescribing studies, perhaps employing structured, multidimensional interventions in contrast to existing discontinuation studies. We acknowledge that this may necessitate novel research methodologies that account for the complexity of the intervention, greater pragmatism of study design and increased focus on patient-centered outcomes. Furthermore, new mechanisms of funding this research may need to be incentivized. When seeking US Food and Drug (FDA) indications, pharmaceutical companies might offer to conduct research and share data and guidelines on how to optimally discontinue (in addition to initiating) a new medication. In the meantime, providers and patients continue to gain clinical and lived experience, respectively, to share in their immediate circles and hopefully beyond.

Case Examples

Case Example 1

Graham's prescriber raises a question around the pros and cons of continuing clozapine, to which Graham agrees to a deprescribing trial. The patient chooses to include his primary clinician (who he meets with weekly), who is initially reluctant to endorse the idea, citing his last inpatient hospitalization 5 years ago when he self-presented with distress around egodystonic command auditory hallucinations to harm others. Nevertheless, considering the uncertainty around the adequacy of past medication trials, potential gains of reduced metabolic side effects and improved related function, collaboration around a structured deprescribing plan (including WRAP) and continued contact with his weekly clozapine group (with whom he has grown very attached), all stakeholders agree to gradually taper the clozapine over 9 months. He remains on the haloperidol 10mg qhs with a provisional agreement to optimize this, in the next instance, if necessary.

Graham begins to steadily lose weight, giving him a newfound enthusiasm for attending the gym and making other lifestyle modifications, leading to further improvements in his cardiovascular risk factors.

Although the frequency of his voices have not increased, at month 5, Graham reports increased distress and difficulty employing his established coping strategies, accompanied by insomnia. A short-term hypnotic is prescribed, and he gains the motivation to attend a Hearing Voices Network meeting (which was previously recommended by a peer and on his deprescribing plan as a potential future self-initiated wellness strategies). At month 7, Graham becomes more internally preoccupied and reports increasing paranoia. At 100 mg total daily clozapine and a serum level less than 150, Graham and his prescriber agree to implement the backup plan to optimize the less metabolically impactful haloperidol (while continuing the planned clozapine taper). Graham agrees to the convenience of a once-a-month haloperidol decanoate depot injection and finally discloses to his prescriber that had actually only been taking his haloperidol tablets intermittently, as needed for sleep. Graham in fact completes the clozapine deprescribing as planned at 9 months; however, the original plan has been adjusted to include attendance of Hearing Voices Network meetings and the addition of intramuscular haloperidol decanoate 100 mg monthly, which he tolerates well (Table 9.5).

Table 9.5 Decision making grid for case 1

Decision-making grid		
	Risks	Benefits
Continuing clozapine	Weight gain	Unclear/Due to poor documentation, the need for clozapine was not clearly established
Deprescribing clozapine	Relapse and rehospitalization	Reduced side effects, more investment in non-pharmacological interventions

Patient values/preference: Patient wishes to reduce and stop clozapine

Plan: Psychoeducation, WRAP, CBT, involvement of any significant others, replacement of clozapine with a medication with a more acceptable side-effect profile; short-term management of symptoms such as insomnia

Interventions: Deprescribe clozapine and replace with haloperidol; WRAP;

Case Example 2

Jane is a 37-year-old woman who was initially prescribed haloperidol 5 mg along with an antidepressant because she was paranoid about people at work staring at her and talking about her. She has never been hospitalized. She still has similar thoughts occasionally but is able to dismiss them. She tells her doctor that she has been well for 2 years and does not want to take medications anymore.

Jane presumably developed persecutory delusions in the context of a depressive episode. In this case, it is appropriate to attempt deprescribing the AP after the depressive episode has subsided (Table 9.6).

Table 9.6 Decision-making grid for case 2

Decision-making grid		
	Risks	Benefits
Continuing haloperidol	Long-term side effects including tardive dyskinesia	Lesser risk of reappearance of paranoia
Deprescribing haloperidol	Reappearance of paranoia	Development of non-pharmacological strategies Patient preference
Patient values/preference: Patient wishes to reduce and stop haloperidol		
Plan: Psychoeducation, WRAP, CBT, involvement of any significant others		
Interventions: Deprescribe haloperidol		

Case Example 3

Tom is a 36-year-old man who carries a diagnosis of schizophrenia but has limited insight. He is prescribed risperidone 4 mg at bedtime, but unbeknownst to his prescriber he only takes it approximately 3–4 times a week. He also smokes daily marijuana and asserts that he doesn't really need the risperidone because the marijuana helps with his anxiety (driven by positive symptoms) much better. Tom also asked about a class action law suit advertised on TV in relation to potential side effects from this medication a month ago. His records reflect that he has not had any hospitalizations related to psychosis since he started taking the AP. Tom presents to the office more agitated than before and demands to stop the risperidone, he demonstrates no positive symptoms or imminent risk.

Tom demonstrates little in the way of buy-in or perceived benefit from risperidone. He admits to having been taking a lesser than prescribed dose and may infact have self-discontinued the medication already. The prescriber suspects that recommending Tom continue the risperidone is unlikely to yield positive results. Instead she maintains a stance of exploration and curiosity to ensure that Tom continues to be engaged. Psychoeducation around the risks of abrupt discontinuation is provided and Tom accepts a gradual taper instead alongside reduction in his marijuana use. By completing the deprescribing worksheet together, it becomes clear that sexual side effects were a big issue for Tom and aripiprazole is agreed upon as an alternative strategy for early warning symptoms (Tom identifies that paranoia drives his anxiety). 2 months pass without AP prescription until Tom calls his prescriber to request initiation of aripiprazole in response to growing paranoia (Table 9.7).

Table 9.7 Decision making grid for case 3

Decision-making grid		
	Risks	Benefits
Continuing risperidone	Long-term side effects, Tom doesn't want to take it	Prevention of rehospitalization
Deprescribing risperidone	Risk of relapse and rehospitalization	Patient preference
Patient values/preference: Patient wants to stop risperidone		
Plan: Continue psychoeducation, further discussion to reach a decision that both doctor and patient can agree on		
Interventions: Psychoeducation, exploration of why he wants to stop the medication		

Self-Assessment

1. Amy has taken haloperidol 10 mg twice a day for more than 30 years. She has severe tardive dyskinesia (TD) and stays home all the time because she is so embarrassed about the involuntary movements. She is asking if reducing the dose of haloperidol will help with the movements. She and you decide to go ahead with reducing the

haloperidol. When Amy's older son hears about this, he leaves a very angry message on your phone, threatening to sue you for reducing the haloperidol.

   a. What will your next steps be?

   b. How will you approach the threat of legal consequences?

   c. Do you think that a reduction in dose may cause an improvement in the TD?

2. Ben is a 40-year-old man who has taken quetiapine and lithium for 3 years, following a severe manic episode in which he lost his entire life savings. He is single and wants to find a partner but won't try because he is ashamed of his weight. He is also concerned about his inability to perform sexually. When you bring up the possibility of reducing quetiapine, he immediately refuses.

   a. How do you understand Ben's reaction?

   b. How will you approach his fear of relapse?

   c. If Ben declines to reduce the quetiapine, what will your next steps be?

References

Anderson, S. L., & Vande Griend, J. P. (2014). Quetiapine for insomnia: A review of the literature. *American Journal of Health System Pharmacology,* *71*(5), 394–402.

Andreasen, N. C., Carpenter Jr, W. T., Kane, J. M., Lasser, R. A., Marder, S. R., & Weinberger, D. R. (2005). Remission in schizophrenia: Proposed criteria and rationale for consensus. *American Journal of Psychiatry, 162*(3), 441–449.

American Psychiatric Association (APA). 2005). *Position Statement on the Use of the Concept of Recovery.* Washington DC: American Psychiatric Association.

American Psychiatric Association (APA). (2006). *American Psychiatric Association Practice Guidelines for the Treatment of Psychiatric Disorders: Compendium.* Washington, DC: American Psychiatric Association.

Barrowclough, C., Haddock, G., Tarrier, N., Lewis, S. W., Moring, J., O'Brien, R., . . . McGovern, J. (2001). Randomized controlled trial of motivational interviewing, cognitive behavior therapy, and family intervention for patients with comorbid schizophrenia and substance use disorders. *American Journal of Psychiatry, 158*(10), 1706–1713.

Bjerre, L. M., Farrell, B., Hogel, M., Graham, L., Lemay, G., McCarthy, L., . . . Welch, V. (2018). Deprescribing antipsychotics for behavioural and psychological symptoms of dementia and insomnia: Evidence-based clinical practice guideline. *Canadian Family Physician, 64*(1), 17–27.

Borlido, C., Remington, G., Graff-Guerrero, A., Arenovich, T., Hazra, M., Wong, A., . . . Mamo, D. C. (2016). Switching from 2 antipsychotics to 1 antipsychotic in schizophrenia: A randomized, double-blind, placebo-controlled study. *Journal of Clinical Psychiatry, 77*(1), 14–20.

Cannon, T. D., Yu, C., Addington, J., Bearden, C. E., Cadenhead, K. S., Cornblatt, B. A., . . . Perkins, D. O. (2016). An individualized risk calculator for research in prodromal psychosis. *American Journal of Psychiatry, 173*(10), 980–988.

Cerovecki, A., Musil, R., Klimke, A., Seemüller, F., Haen, E., Schennach, R., . . . Riedel, M. (2013). Withdrawal symptoms and rebound syndromes associated with switching and discontinuing atypical antipsychotics: Theoretical background and practical recommendations. *CNS Drugs, 27*(7), 545–572.

Chen, E. Y., Hui, C. L., Lam, M. M., Chiu, C. P., Law, C. W., Chung, D. W., . . . Mo, F. Y. (2010). Maintenance treatment with quetiapine versus discontinuation after one year of treatment in patients with remitted first episode psychosis: Randomised controlled trial. *British Medical Journal, 341*: c4024.

Chouinard, G. (1991). Severe cases of neuroleptic-induced supersensitivity psychosis: Diagnostic criteria for the disorder and its treatment. *Schizophrenia Research, 5*(1), 21–33.

Chouinard, G., & V.-A. Chouinard (2008). Atypical antipsychotics: CATIE study, drug-induced movement disorder and resulting iatrogenic psychiatric-like symptoms, supersensitivity rebound psychosis and withdrawal discontinuation syndromes. *Psychotherapy and Psychosomatics, 77*(2), 69–77.

Coe, H. V., & I. S. Hong (2012). Safety of low doses of quetiapine when used for insomnia. *Annals of Pharmacotherapy, 46*(5), 718–722.

Copeland, M. E. (1997). *Wellness Recovery Action Plan*. Brattleboro, VT: Peach Press.

Corstens, D., Longden, E., McCarthy-Jones, S., Waddingham, R., & Thomas, N. (2014). Emerging perspectives from the Hearing Voices Movement: Implications for research and practice. *Schizophrenia Bulletin, 40*(Suppl 4), S285–S294.

Drake, R. E., O'Neal, E. L., & Wallach, M. A. (2008). A systematic review of psychosocial research on psychosocial interventions for people with co-occurring severe mental and substance use disorders. *Journal of Substance Abuse Treatment, 34*(1), 123–138.

Dufresne, R. L., & Wagner, R., L. (1988). Antipsychotic-withdrawal akathisia versus antipsychotic-induced akathisia: Further evidence for the existence of tardive akathisia. *Journal of Clinical Psychiatry, 49*(11), 435–438.

Essock, S. M., Covell, N. H., Leckman-Westin, E., Lieberman, J. A., Sederer, L. I., Kealey, E., & Finnerty, M. T. (2009). Identifying clinically questionable psychotropic prescribing practices for Medicaid recipients in New York State. *Psychiatric Services, 60*(12), 1595–1602.

Falloon, I. R., Boyd, J. L., McGill, C. W., Razani, J., Moss, H. B., & Gilderman, A. M. (1982). Family management in the prevention of exacerbations of schizophrenia: A controlled study. *New England Journal of Medicine, 306*(24), 1437–1440.

Findling, R. L., Steiner, H., & Weller, E. B. (2004). Use of antipsychotics in children and adolescents. *Journal of Clinical Psychiatry, 66*, 29–40.

Ganguly, R., Kotzan, J. A., Miller, L. S., Kennedy, K., & Martin, B. C. (2004). Prevalence, trends, and factors associated with antipsychotic polypharmacy among Medicaid-eligible schizophrenia patients, 1998–2000. *Journal of Clinical Psychiatry, 65*(10), 1377–1388.

Gilbert, P. L., Harris, M. J., McAdams, L. A., & Jeste, D. V.(1995). Neuroleptic withdrawal in schizophrenic patients: A review of the literature. *Archives of General Psychiatry, 52*(3), 173–188.

Goff, D. C., Falkai, P., Fleischhacker, W. W., Girgis, R. R., Kahn, R. M., Uchida, H., . . . Lieberman, J. A. (2017). The long-term effects of antipsychotic medication on clinical course in schizophrenia. *American Journal of Psychiatry, 174*(9), 840–849.

Gordon, C., Gidugu, V., Rogers, E. S., DeRonck, J., & Ziedonis, D. (2016). Adapting open dialogue for early-onset psychosis into the US health care environment: A feasibility study. *Psychiatric Services, 67*(11), 1166–1168.

Harrow, M., & Jobe, T., H. (2013). Does long-term treatment of schizophrenia with antipsychotic medications facilitate recovery? *Schizophrenia Bulletin, 39*(5), 962–965.

Hasan, A., Falkai, P., Wobrock, T., Lieberman, J., Glenthoj, B., Gattaz, W. F., . . . WFSBP Task Force on Treatment Guidelines for Schizophrenia. (2012). World Federation of Societies of Biological Psychiatry (WFSBP) Guidelines for Biological Treatment of Schizophrenia, part 1: Update 2012 on the acute treatment of schizophrenia and the management of treatment resistance. *World Journal of Biological Psychiatry, 13*(5), 318–378.

Hermes, E., Sernyak, M., & Rosenheck, R. (2014). The use of second generation antipsychotics for post-traumatic stress disorder in a US Veterans Health Administration Medical Center. *Epidemiology and Psychiatric Sciences, 23*(03), 281–288.

Hogarty, G. E., Anderson, C. M., Reiss, D. J., Kornblith, S. J., Greenwald, D. P., Ulrich, R. F., & Carter, M. (1991). Family psychoeducation, social skills training, and maintenance chemotherapy in the aftercare treatment of schizophrenia: II. Two-year effects of a controlled study on relapse and adjustment. *Archives of General Psychiatry, 48*(4), 340–347.

Katona, L., Czobor, P., & Bitter, I. (2014). Real-world effectiveness of antipsychotic monotherapy vs. polypharmacy in schizophrenia: To switch or to combine? A nationwide study in Hungary. *Schizophrenia Research, 152*(1), 246–254.

Kreyenbuhl, J., Buchanan, R. W., Dickerson, F. B., & Dixon, L. B. (2010). The schizophrenia patient outcomes research team (PORT), updated treatment recommendations 2009. *Schizophrenia Bulletin, 36*(1), 94–103.

Lacoursiere, R. B., Spohn, H. E., & Thompson, K. (1976). Medical effects of abrupt neuroleptic withdrawal. *Comprehensive Psychiatry, 17*(2), 285–294.

Leucht, S., Tardy, M., Komossa, K., Heres, S., Kissling, W., Salanti, G., & Davis, J. M. (2012). Antipsychotic drugs versus placebo for relapse prevention in schizophrenia: A systematic review and meta-analysis. *Lancet, 379*(9831), 2063–2071.

McFarlane, W. R., Dixon, L., Lukens, E., & Lucksted, A. (2003). Family psychoeducation and schizophrenia: A review of the literature. *Journal of Marital and Family Therapy, 29*(2), 223–245.

McGurk, S. R., Twamley, E. W., Sitzer, D. I., McHugo, G. J., & Mueser, K. T. (2007). A meta-analysis of cognitive remediation in schizophrenia. *American Journal of Psychiatry, 164*(12), 1791–1802.

Moncrieff, J. (2006). Does antipsychotic withdrawal provoke psychosis? Review of the literature on rapid onset psychosis (supersensitivity psychosis) and withdrawal-related relapse. *Acta Psychiatrica Scandinavica, 114*(1), 3–13.

Murray, R. M. (2016). Mistakes I have made in my research career. *Schizophrenia Bulletin*. sbw165.

Murray, R. M., Quattrone, D., Natesan, S., van Os, J., Nordentoft, M., Howes, O., . . . Taylor, D. (2016). (2016). Should psychiatrists be more cautious about the long-term prophylactic use of antipsychotics? *British Journal of Psychiatry, 209*(5), 361–365.

Park, S. Y., Cervesi, C., Galling, B., Molteni, S., Walyzada, F., Ameis, S. H., . . . Correll, C. U. (2016). Antipsychotic use trends in youth with autism spectrum disorder and/or intellectual disability: A meta-analysis. *Journal of the American Academy of Child & Adolescent Psychiatry, 55*(6), 456–468. e454.

Petrakis, I. L., Nich, C., & Ralevski, E. (2006). Psychotic spectrum disorders and alcohol abuse: A review of pharmacotherapeutic strategies and a report on the effectiveness of naltrexone and disulfiram. *Schizophrenia Bulletin, 32*(4), 644–654.

Pilling, S., Bebbington, P., Kuipers, E., Garety, P., Geddes, J., Orbach, G., & Morgan, C. (2002). Psychological treatments in schizophrenia: I. Meta-analysis of family intervention and cognitive behaviour therapy. *Psychological Medicine, 32*(05), 763–782.

Saha, S., Chant, D., & McGrath, J. (2007). A systematic review of mortality in schizophrenia: Is the differential mortality gap worsening over time? *Archives of General Psychiatry, 64*(10), 1123–1131.

Seikkula, B. A., Jukka, A., J. (2001). Open dialogue in psychosis II: A comparison of good and poor outcome cases. *Journal of Constructivist Psychology, 14*(4), 267–284.

Stahl, S., & Grady, M. (2004). A critical review of atypical antipsychotic utilization: Comparing monotherapy with polypharmacy and augmentation. *Current Medicinal Chemistry, 11*(3), 313–327.

Swofford, C. D., Kasckow, J. W., Scheller-Gilkey, G., & Inderbitzin, L. B. (1996). Substance use: A powerful predictor of relapse in schizophrenia. *Schizophrenia Research, 20*(1), 145–151.

Takeuchi, H., Kantor, N., Uchida, H., Suzuki, T., & Remington, G. (2017). Immediate vs gradual discontinuation in antipsychotic switching: A systematic review and meta-analysis. *Schizophrenia Bulletin, 43*(4), 862–871.

Takeuchi, H., Suzuki, T., Uchida, H., Watanabe, K., & Mimura, M. (2012). Antipsychotic treatment for schizophrenia in the maintenance phase: A systematic review of the guidelines and algorithms. *Schizophrenia Research, 134*(2), 219–225.

Thaker, G. K., Wagman, A. M., Kirkpatrick, B., & Tamminga, C. A. (1989). Alterations in sleep polygraphy after neuroleptic withdrawal: A putative supersensitive dopaminergic mechanism. *Biological Psychiatry, 25*(1), 75–86.

Tiihonen, J., Tanskanen, A., & Taipale, H. (2018). 20-year nationwide follow-up study on discontinuation of antipsychotic treatment in first-episode schizophrenia. *American Journal of Psychiatry*, appi-ajp.

Viguera, A. C., Baldessarini, R. J., Hegarty, J. D., van Kammen, D. P., & Tohen, M. (1997). Clinical risk following abrupt and gradual withdrawal of maintenance neuroleptic treatment. *Archives of General Psychiatry, 54*(1), 49–55.

Wunderink, L., Nieboer, R. M., Wiersma, D., Sytema, S., & Nienhuis, F. J. (2013). Recovery in remitted first-episode psychosis at 7 years of follow-up of an early dose reduction/discontinuation or maintenance treatment strategy: Long-term follow-up of a 2-year randomized clinical trial. *JAMA Psychiatry, 70*(9), 913–920.

Wunderink, L., Nienhuis, F. J., Sytema, S., Slooff, C. J., Knegtering, R., & Wiersma, D. (2007). Guided discontinuation versus maintenance treatment in remitted first-episode psychosis: Relapse rates and functional outcome. *Journal of Clinical Psychiatry, 68*(5), 654–661.

Zipursky, R. B., Menezes, N. M., & Streiner, D. L. (2014). Risk of symptom recurrence with medication discontinuation in first-episode psychosis: A systematic review. *Schizophrenia Research, 152*(2), 408–414.

10

Deprescribing Mood Stabilizers

In this chapter, we present specific context, considerations and clinical decision-making relevant to deprescribing mood stabilizers, particularly in the treatment of bipolar disorder. We apply the same caveats found in the introduction to chapter 8 and trust the reader will consider the discussion through their own critical lens of knowledge, experience and expertise. Again, deprescribing interventions in this class will include the pursuit of minimum effective dosing as well as complete discontinuation when appropriate. Issues of shared decision making and informed consent are again pertinent when dealing with vulnerable populations such as those experiencing serious mental illnesses. Some distinguishing challenges of deprescribing for bipolar disorder are addressed, along with specific adjunctive strategies.

Goals and Learning Objectives

After reading this chapter, the reader will be able to:

1. Describe three scenarios where deprescribing of mood stabilizers may be appropriate
2. List the particular considerations when deprescribing lithium (in correctly diagnosed bipolar disorder) and how the risks may be mitigated
3. Complete a formal risk–benefit analysis for deprescribing a mood stabilizer in a given patient

Case Example

Jane is a 36-year-old woman who was diagnosed as having schizoaffective disorder in her early 20s. She suffered from what she described as "anger attacks" and mood swings with premenstrual worsening. She was first hospitalized at age 21 with a mixed affective episode during which she heard voices telling her to kill herself. This occurred following the death of a beloved childhood pet. She often hears her name called when "stressed out", however full positive symptoms have only fleetingly presented at the extremes of her mood episodes. She has been in individual therapy and has consistently taken carbamazepine for more than a decade with intermittent use of risperidone. She estimates that she takes about a third of the prescribed risperidone standing bedtime doses, and only when she notices her thoughts racing and "spiraling" and her mood being more irritable. She says that she has gained a better understanding of her mood fluctuations over the years and how to manage them by adjusting her work schedule or soliciting help from her significant other. She wishes to stop taking all medications. Historically, the most significant improvement in symptom management occurred when she moved out of her parents' home 2 years ago.

Arguably Jane, warrants a re-formulation and possible 'undiagnosing' intervention before exploring a deprescribing intervention. It is unlikely that she suffers from a primary psychotic disorder given only spotty psychotic, and more prominent affective, symptoms. Furthermore, the improvement with therapy and altering her social environment demonstrates a significant interpersonal and psychological component to her condition. Jane is well supported by her significant other and her therapist, and is a candidate for deprescribing carbamazepine. She agrees however around continuing the risperidone as needed. The dose of as-needed risperidone is lowered as the carbamazepine is stopped (due to loss of enzyme induction; see Table 10.1). In the course of an increased non-pharmacological focus during medication visits, Jane eventually discloses to her prescriber that she suffered chronic sexual abuse as a child.

Table 10.1 Commonly prescribed mood stabilizers

Medication	Common indications
Lithium	Bipolar spectrum disorders
Lamotrigine	Mood instability in personality disorders
Divalproex	Schizoaffective disorder
Carbamazepine	Augmentation in depressive disorders
	Schizophrenia

Potential Factors Contributing to the Extended Use of Mood Stabilizers

Deprescribing of mood stabilizers may involve a careful review of history and diagnosis before a reestimation of the risk/benefit calculation. Limitations surrounding clinical documentation, retrospective report, high rates of cooccuring substance use and lack of diagnostic tests can thwart the retrospective confirmation of a diagnosis of bipolar disorder. While the effectiveness of mood stabilizers is well-established in correctly diagnosed bipolar disorder, there is perhaps less certain evidence for their use in schizoaffective disorder, in the augmentation of antipsychotic and antidepressant regimens, and in control of mood lability in the context of personality traits or disorders. Mood stabilizers as augmenting agents (especially lithium for major depressive disorder and valproate for psychotic disorders) have no recommendation for the duration of use in these cases. Patients may continue to take these agents indefinitely and without any clear indication because the only way to establish their ongoing need is by evaluating how a patient does without them. Some critics question an 'overdiagnosis' of bipolar disorder which emerged in the 1990s (in turn increasing the risk of over prescription of mood stabilizers). Substance-induced mood disorders, affective instability and impulsivity in personality disorders, and the expansion of the "bipolar spectrum" of disorders are some of the potential driving factors (see Ghouse, Sanches, Zunta-Soares, Swann, & Soares, 2013; Zimmerman, Ruggero, Chelminski, & Young, 2008).

In bipolar disorder, the use of combinations of mood stabilizers has become increasingly common and is recommended by some standard guidelines, in particular those by the American Psychiatric Association (APA, 2006). Mood stabilizers may be prescribed in combination with second-generation antipsychotic medications, which are themselves used as mood stabilizers. In both these situations, the duration of need for combination treatments is uncertain.

Balancing the high risk of mortality and morbidity inherent in untreated bipolar disorder, the commonly prescribed mood stablizers, lithium and divalproex for example, are known to carry risk of potentially serious and persisting neurological, renal, and hepatic side effects. In patients with medical comorbidities that affect renal or hepatic function (e.g. diabetes, hypertension, chronic hepatitis due to various etiologies), these medications may need to be adjusted or eventually discontinued due to evolving medical factors. Several common mood stabilizers (lithium, divalproex and carbamazepine) have routine bloodwork monitoring including drug levels built into the accepted guidelines. The prescriber therefore has the tools and imperative to remain vigilant for changes where a reduction and or discontinuation of mood stabilizers may be warranted or unavoidable.

Lithium

Lithium has established efficacy in preventing relapses of (particularly euphoric) mania in bipolar disorder although its efficacy in preventing bipolar depressive episodes is equivocal (see Geddes, Burgess, Hawton, Jamison, & Goodwin, 2004). Although lithium is used to augment antidepressant treatment of unipolar major depression (Bauer & Döpfmer, 1999), guidelines for the duration of use and expected consequences of discontinuation in this scenario have not been as thoroughly explored for this indication.

Antiepileptic Agents

Coincident with the construction of the expanded 'bipolar spectrum' of disorders and the kindling theory of recurrence, the use of divalproex (introduced in 1995) and lamotrigine (introduced in 1994) exploded (see Akiskal et al., 2000). Both these medications began to be used for the treatment of bipolar disorder, especially type II, either singly, in combination, or in combination with lithium. Divalproex is used for the rapid control of agitation which may stem from a range of etiologies on inpatient psychiatric units (see Deltito, Levitan, Damore, Hajal, & Zambenedetti, 1998). Divalproex does not require the same slow titration to an effective dose as lamotrigine, it acts faster than lithium, and hence it is often preferred in acute settings. Divalproex may offer addition appeal when added to neuroleptic agents to augment their acute tranquilizing effect, and to facilitate quick discharge for inpatient units for example. However, the onus then falls to the outpatient service to re-evaluate (or perhaps decipher) the original indication for the use of divalproex, making it a potential target for deprescribing. A related scenario occurs when a patient experiencing a psychotic episode is prematurely discharged from an inpatient service as the sedation induced by divalproex makes them appear calmer. The underlying psychotic symptoms remain inadequately treated, and when divalproex is then deprescribed on the outpatient service, a florid underlying psychosis may emerge. This scenario highlights the need for careful consideration, timing and planning of a deprescribing even in the face of the most compelling of indications.

Divalproex, lamotrigine, topiramate, zonisamide, and gabapentin are being used increasingly for the management of *alcohol withdrawal* (in lieu of benzodiazepines) as well as *alcohol use disorders* (see Hammond, Niciu, Drew, & Arias, 2015). For alcohol withdrawal, it is intuitive that the medication be tapered off after the risk for withdrawal-related seizures has passed. Unfortunately this literature does not yet specify clear, evidence-based guidelines for duration of treatment.

Lithium Discontinuation Syndromes

There is an extensive literature on relapses, both manic and depressive, precipitated by withdrawal of lithium. For example, as early as 1970, Baastrup and colleagues (1970) noted that both bipolar patients and patients with 'endogenous depression' relapsed following lithium discontinuation. Symptoms of lithium discontinuation typically include physical symptoms such as tremor, polyuria, muscular weakness, polydipsia, and dryness of mouth. However, reported psychiatric relapses (within 4 days of lithium discontinuation), supports the possibility of a *rebound* phenomenon (see Christodoulou & Lykouras, 1982). A review of 10 studies of lithium discontinuation in bipolar disorder concluded that lithium discontinuation "increased the risk of recurrence which may exceed that predicted by the course of the preceding untreated bipolar disorder" (Suppes, Baldessarini, Faedda, & Tohen, 1991). A systematic review and meta-analysis concluded that the odds ratio for a recurrence following an interruption in lithium treatment was 1.4 compared to continuous treatment (Vries et al., 2013). Studies have also identified increased daytime motor activity (Klein, Lavie, Meiraz, Sadeh, & Lenox, 1992) and changes in the sleep–wake cycle (Klein, Mairaz, Pascal, Hefez, & Lavie, 1991) as early signs of relapse following lithium discontinuation. Even patients who did not relapse experienced anxiety, nervousness, increased irritability, alertness, sleep disturbances, and occasionally an elated mood beginning several days after lithium discontinuation and lasting 1–2 weeks (Klein et al., 1991). When lithium is used as an augmenting agent in major depression, one study found that, in older individuals with major depression, abrupt cessation of lithium could precipitate a depressive relapse (Fahy & Lawlor, 2001). This was followed by a systematic review of three articles that reached a similar conclusion (Ross, 2008).

Reports like these provide sufficient doubt to question whether the relapses following lithium discontinuation are a recurrence of the underlying illness or a withdrawal phenomenon. As the definitive mechanism of action of lithium remains unknown, any theories about the neurobiological basis of lithium withdrawal are speculative. Dopamine supersensitivity, cellular transport, and membrane changes are some putative mechanisms and have been demonstrated in small animal studies (see Balon, Yeragani, Pohl, & Gershon, 1988). Another reported concern surrounding lithium discontinuation is that when restarted for a given patient, lithium would cease to be as effective as it had originally been—a mechanism for this has not been established.

It is therefore warranted to determine if the risk of relapse following lithium discontinuation can be mitigated by slowing the rate of taper. Interestingly, studies found that the early risk as well as the overall 5-year risk of recurrence was lower following gradual discontinuation (e.g. over 2–4 weeks) as compared to rapid taper (e.g. less than 2 weeks; see Faedda, Tondo, Baldessarini, Suppes, & Tohen, 1993, Baldessarini et al., 1996; Baldessarini, Tondo, Floris, & Rudas, 1997).

Some Considerations when Deprescribing Mood Stabilizers

The deprescribing of antiepileptic drugs (AEDs) prescribed for psychiatric indications has not yet been studied systematically. The only literature currently available is from discontinuation studies conducted in patients with epilepsy (using seizure recurrences as the main outcome, and not commenting on mood disturbances or sleep for example). A literature review of AED discontinuation in patients with epilepsy (Vernachio, Lovett, & Williams, 2015) states that tapering schedules varied widely (ranging from 4 days to 4 years) and that although there was a general agreement that AED discontinuation needed to be considered, there was no consensus on which patients for whom it would be indicated. A single case report describes a manic episode precipitated by carbamazepine withdrawal in a woman with epilepsy (Scull & Trimble, 1995).

The process of deprecribing (as with prescribing) involves careful consideration of drug-drug interactions and consultation with pharmacy as needed. One example is the loss of CP450 enzyme induction when deprescribing. A case report describes the development of parkinsonian symptoms after discontinuation of carbamazepine in a patient who was taking a combination of risperidone and carbamazepine (see Takahashi, Yoshida, Higuchi, & Shimizu, 2001). Monitoring for emergence of extrapyramidal symptoms has been recommended when carbamazepine is discontinued in patients who are taking concomitant antipsychotic medications that are a CYP3A4 substrate (Strack, Leckband, & Meyer, 2009). A review of AED discontinuation in patients with epilepsy cites several case reports of withdrawal symptoms such as akathisia, agitation, nausea, insomnia, abdominal pain, and anxiety following the abrupt withdrawal of high doses of gabapentin (see Vernachio et al., 2015).

Non-pharmacological Strategies to Support Deprescribing of Mood Stabilizers

So far, psychotherapeutic interventions have been relegated to adjunctive treatments in bipolar disorder, and there are very few data to support the use of such interventions as the primary modality of treatment. A review of psychotherapeutic interventions in bipolar disorder found that adjunctive family therapy, interpersonal therapy, and systematic care improved outcomes immediately in an acute episode, whereas cognitive behavior therapy (CBT) and group psychoeducation were more effective in improving functioning and reducing rates of relapse (Miklowitz, 2008). Psychoeducation, CBT, interpersonal and social rhythms therapy, and family interventions are commonly tested treatments both in short- and long-term studies, are feasible for patients with more complex bipolar disorder (see Reinares, Sánchez-Moreno, & Fountoulakis, 2014).

One small, but illuminating, qualitative study describes the decision-making surrounding mood stabilizers and the strategies that patients use to keep themselves well without medications. The authors developed a model in the form of a sequential process that is influenced by the concept of "ideas about myself and my moods." Strategies were highly individual and ranged from "taking time off work" to "lighting scented oils" for example (see Cappleman, Smith, & Lobban, 2015). Further strategies and ideas for additional non-pharmacological strategies are described in Chapters 5 and 6.

Conclusion

The predominant literature available to guide the pharmacological aspects of deprescribing mood stabilizers in psychiatry comes from lithium discontinuation studies conducted between 1970 and 1990 and points to the possible existence of a lithium withdrawal syndrome that may be independent of recurrence of the underlying bipolar disorder. No guidelines and limited studies are currently available to inform the safe withdrawal of AEDs when used as mood stabilizers.

Case Examples

Case Example 1

Joe, a 30-year-old man has been taking aripiprazole 20 mg/d along with divalproex ER 1,500 mg at night for the past 4 months. These medications were prescribed at his first hospitalization, in which he believed with delusional intensity that he was a famous actor and was irritable and angry. He quickly returned to his usual state of health and experiences no side effects except for some daytime sleepiness. He tolerates the sedation, and has returned to work.

The current formulation is that Joe experienced a first episode of psychosis (with mania-like features) that could differentiate into either primary bipolar disorder or schizophrenia. In either case, aripiprazole was indicated to treat the episode and might provide some prophylaxis of further episodes (affective or psychotic). There is currently unclear indication for or benefit from continuation of divalproex. Even if a clear indication such as the need for augmentation of aripiprazole was identifiable, there is no guideline for how long divalproex should be continued as an augmenting agent. As Joe is not actively inquiring about deprescribing, a first step in this case would be to opening explain the risks and benefits of continued divalproex and obtain his opinion (see Table 10.2). With this initial discussion in place, there may be no urgency to make a change in the regimen.

Table 10.2 Example Decision-making grid for case 2

Decision-making grid		
	Risks	Benefits
Continuing lithium	Nephrotoxicity Neurotoxicity	Prevention of manic and depressive episodes
Deprescribing lithium	Mania or depression Suicidality Possible treatment refractoriness	Removes long-term risks of lithium

Patient values/preference: Patient has expressed an interest in discontinuing lithium

Plan: Explore reasons for enquiring about discontinuation; discuss risks and benefits of stopping lithium; provide alternate medication strategies

Intervention: Switch to another medication; offer psychoeducation on early identification of relapse; develop a plan for management of suicidality if it emerges during lithium discontinuation; slow taper of lithium; plan for resumption of lithium if needed

Case Example 2

Jack, a 45-year-old man has been taking lithium for more than 15 years for a diagnosis of bipolar 1 disorder. It was started when he was hospitalized for a manic episode in his late 20s. Since then, he has had brief periods of hypomania and two depressive episodes, but none warranting hospitalization. He experiences no side effects other than a fine hand tremor. He states, "I have done my time" and is asking for your opinion on discontinuing lithium.

Guidelines dictate that lithium should be continued indefinitely, especially since there is demonstrable benefit. However, if the patient is asking about discontinuation, this should be addressed by exploring the reason for the inquiry. If it is due to side effects, this may be resolved by dose adjustments or other strategies. If he wishes to begin a trial without lithium, it will need to be tapered slowly with supervision and support from the care team to minimize chances of relapse (and missed opportunity for alternative wellness strategies) that might occur if he initiates a discontinuation on his own.

The prescriber may find themselves pulled in two opposite directions in this scenario—a duty to follow standard professional guidelines, thereby reducing the perceived risk of relapse, and another: to respect the patient's autonomy and perhaps even "right to fail." The prescriber must remember that this tension is never fully resolved, whatever action they eventually recommend. Rather than resolution, the prescriber's responsibility in such a situation is to build tolerance for this tension, perhaps even to maintain it as they work with the patient. They must also have honest discussions with the patient about justified concerns regarding relapse and respect for the patient's autonomy. This will hopefully reduce the chances that Jack will abruptly discontinue lithium without telling the prescriber and will foster the therapeutic alliance. At the same time, it is important to acknowledge that Jack may very well relapse even while continuing to take lithium and that it may not be the only factor in his life that is preventing a relapse (see Table 10.3).

Table 10.3 Example Decision-making grid for case 2

Decision-making grid		
	Risks	Benefits
Continuing lithium	Nephrotoxicity Neurotoxicity	Prevention of manic and depressive episodes
Deprescribing lithium	Mania or depression Suicidality Possible treatment refractoriness	Removes long-term risks of lithium

Patient values/preference: Patient has expressed an interest in discontinuing lithium

Plan: Explore reasons for enquiring about discontinuation; discuss risks and benefits of stopping lithium; provide alternate medication strategies

Intervention: Switch to another medication; offer psychoeducation on early identification of relapse; develop a plan for management of suicidality if it emerges during lithium discontinuation; slow taper of lithium; plan for resumption of lithium if needed

Case Example 3

Hamid is a 65-year-old man who was diagnosed with bipolar disorder in his early 20s. He has taken lithium since then and has had three admissions for manic episodes and persistent low-grade depressive symptoms thereafter. Quetiapine was added at a recent admission. He however experience an episode of lithium toxicity soon after, ending up in the ICU. He says "this medication very nearly killed me. I am never going to take it again." See Table 10.4. The challenge here is to first acknowledge and process the potentially traumatic event before attempting to engage around a more balanced weighing of risks and benefits of the medication regimen. Buy-in may be able to build around the quetiapine as an alternative mood stabilizer.

Table 10.4 Example Decision-making grid for case 3

Decision-making grid		
	Risks	Benefits
Continuing lithium	Long-term side effects such as nephrotoxicity	Prevention of future episodes of mania or depression
Deprescribing lithium	Recurrence of episodes	Removes long-term risks Hamid refuses to take lithium anymore

Patient values/preference: Patient wants to discontinue lithium

Plan: Further discussion about risks and benefits with Hamid. If he continues to reduce lithium, plan on increasing quetiapine to the dose of a primary mood stabilizer

Intervention: Offer psychoeducation on early identification of relapse; develop a plan for management of suicidality if it emerges during lithium discontinuation; slow taper of lithium; plan for resumption of lithium if needed

Self-Assessment

1. Prakash is 25-year-old-man who has taken lithium since he was 16. He says that because he doesn't use drugs anymore, he doesn't need to take lithium and is asking for your help to stop it.
   a. How will you approach Prakash's request?
   b. What are your fears about reducing the lithium?
   c. What will you recommend to minimize the risk of recurrence?

2. Jane is a 30-year-old woman who was prescribed divalproex on the inpatient service, where she was admitted for severe depression and anxiety. She says it helps her sleep but has caused marked hair loss. She refuses to take it anymore.
   a. What might be the indications for prescribing divalproex in this case?
   b. What are your concerns in deprescribing divalproex in this case?
   c. How will you allay your own concerns if you help Jane reduce divalproex?

3. Maritza is a 45-year-old woman admitted for treatment of alcohol withdrawal. She is detoxed from alcohol using gabapentin and discharged on a dose of 800 mg three times a day. Four weeks later during a follow-up, she says she is sleepy and gaining weight but doesn't feel like drinking as much as before. She is asking for your opinion about the gabapentin.
   a. What would you suggest to Maritza in this case?
   b. What would be your concerns in continuing gabapentin?
   c. What would be your concerns in deprescribing gabapentin?

References

Akiskal, H. S., Bourgeois, M. L., Angst, J., Post, R., Möller, H.-J., & Hirschfeld, R. (2000). Re-evaluating the prevalence of and diagnostic composition within the broad clinical spectrum of bipolar disorders. *Journal of Affective Disorders, 59*, S5–S30.

APA. (2006). *American Psychiatric Association Practice Guidelines for the Treatment of Psychiatric Disorders: Compendium 2006*. Washington, DC: American Psychiatric Publishers.

Baastrup, P., Poulsen, J., Schou, M., Thomsen, K., & Amdisen, A. (1970). Prophylactic lithium: Double blind discontinuation in manic-depressive and recurrent-depressive disorders. *Lancet, 296*(7668), 326–330.

Baldessarini, R. J., Tondo, L., Faedda, G. L., Suppes, T. R., Floris, G., & Rudas, N. (1996). Effects of the rate of discontinuing lithium maintenance treatment in bipolar disorders. *Journal of Clinical Psychiatry, 57*(10), 441–448.

Baldessarini, R. J., Tondo, L., Floris, G., & Rudas, N. (1997). Reduced morbidity after gradual discontinuation of lithium treatment for bipolar I and II disorders: A replication study. *American Journal of Psychiatry, 154*(4), 551.

Balon, R., Yeragani, V. K., Pohl, R. B., & Gershon, S. (1988). Lithium discontinuation: Withdrawal or relapse? *Comprehensive Psychiatry*, *29*(3), 330–334.

Bauer, M., & Döpfmer, S. (1999). Lithium augmentation in treatment-resistant depression: Meta-analysis of placebo-controlled studies. *Journal of Clinical Psychopharmacology*, *19*(5), 427–434.

Cappleman, R., Smith, I., & Lobban, F. (2015). Managing bipolar moods without medication: A qualitative investigation. *Journal of Affective Disorders*, *174*, 241–249.

Christodoulou, G., & Lykouras, E. (1982). Abrupt lithium discontinuation in manic-depressive patients. *Acta Psychiatrica Scandinavica*, *65*(5), 310–314.

Deltito, J., Levitan, J., Damore, J., Hajal, F., & Zambenedetti, M. (1998). Naturalistic experience with the use of divalproex sodium on an in-patient unit for adolescent psychiatric patients. *Acta Psychiatrica Scandinavica*, *97*(3), 236–240.

Faedda, G. L., Tondo, L., Baldessarini, R. J., Suppes, T., & Tohen, M. (1993). Outcome after rapid vs gradual discontinuation of lithium treatment in bipolar disorders. *Archives of General Psychiatry*, *50*(6), 448–455.

Fahy, S., & Lawlor, B. A. (2001). Discontinuation of lithium augmentation in an elderly cohort. *International Journal of Geriatric Psychiatry*, *16*(10), 1004–1009.

Geddes, J. R., Burgess, S., Hawton, K., Jamison, K., & Goodwin, G. M. (2004). Long-term lithium therapy for bipolar disorder: Systematic review and meta-analysis of randomized controlled trials. *American Journal of Psychiatry*, *161*(2), 217–222.

Ghouse, A. A., Sanches, M., Zunta-Soares, G., Swann, A. C., & Soares, J. C. (2013). Overdiagnosis of bipolar disorder: A critical analysis of the literature. *Scientific World Journal* vol. 2013, Article ID 297087, 5 pages, 2013. https://doi.org/10.1155/2013/297087.

Hammond, C. J., Niciu, M. J., Drew, S., & Arias, A. J. (2015). Anticonvulsants for the treatment of alcohol withdrawal syndrome and alcohol use disorders. *CNS Drugs*, *29*(4), 293–311.

Klein, E., Lavie, P., Meiraz, R., Sadeh, A., & Lenox, R. (1992). Increased motor activity and recurrent manic episodes: Predictors of rapid relapse in remitted bipolar disorder patients after lithium discontinuation. *Biological Psychiatry*, *31*(3), 279–284.

Klein, E., Mairaz, R., Pascal, M., Hefez, A., & Lavie, P. (1991). Discontinuation of lithium treatment in remitted bipolar patients: Relationship between clinical outcome and changes in sleep-wake cycles. *Journal of Nervous and Mental Disease*, *179*(8), 499–501.

Miklowitz, D. J. (2008). Adjunctive psychotherapy for bipolar disorder: State of the evidence. *American Journal of Psychiatry, 165*(11), 1408–1419.

Reinares, M., Sánchez-Moreno, J., & Fountoulakis, K. N. (2014). Psychosocial interventions in bipolar disorder: What, for whom, and when. *Journal of Affective Disorders, 156*, 46–55.

Ross, J. (2008). Discontinuation of lithium augmentation in geriatric patients with unipolar depression: A systematic review. *Canadian Journal of Psychiatry, 53*(2), 117–120.

Scull, D., & Trimble, M. (1995). Mania precipitated by carbamazepine withdrawal. *British Journal of Psychiatry, 167*(5), 698.

Strack, D. K., Leckband, S. G., & Meyer, J. M. (2009). Antipsychotic prescribing practices following withdrawal of concomitant carbamazepine. *Journal of Psychiatric Practice, 15*(6), 442–448.

Suppes, T., Baldessarini, R. J., Faedda, G. L., & Tohen, M. (1991). Risk of recurrence following discontinuation of lithium treatment in bipolar disorder. *Archives of General Psychiatry, 48*(12), 1082–1088.

Takahashi, H., Yoshida, K., Higuchi, H., & Shimizu, T. (2001). Development of parkinsonian symptoms after discontinuation of carbamazepine in patients concurrently treated with risperidone: Two case reports. *Clinical Neuropharmacology, 24*(6), 358–360.

Vernachio, K., Lovett, A., & Williams, J. (2015). A review of withdraw strategies for discontinuing antiepileptic therapy in epilepsy and pain management. *Pharmacy and Pharmacology International Journal, 3*(1), 00045.

Vries, C., Bergen, A., Regeer, E. J., Benthem, E., Kupka, R. W., & Boks, M. P. (2013). The effectiveness of restarted lithium treatment after discontinuation: Reviewing the evidence for discontinuation-induced refractoriness. *Bipolar Disorders, 15*(6), 645–649.

Zimmerman, M., Ruggero, C. J., Chelminski, I., & Young, D. (2008). Is bipolar disorder overdiagnosed? *Journal of Clinical Psychiatry, 69*(6), 935–940.

11

Deprescribing Benzodiazepines, Z-Drugs, and Stimulants

This chapter frames challenges and discusses strategies for deprescribing medications that may exhibit habit forming/rewarding properties, and hence additional investment in continuing or difficulty discontinuing may exist for the patient. Medications that we will be discussing include BZDs, the z-drugs (zolpidem, zopiclone, eszopiclone, and zaleplon), and stimulant medications used to treat attention deficit hyperactivity disorder (ADHD) such as methylphenidate (e.g. Ritalin), methylphenidate extended release (e.g. Concerta), dexmethylphenidate (e.g. Focalin), mixed amphetamine salts (e.g. Adderall), and lisdexamphetamine (e.g. Vyvanse). The same issues of shared decision making and informed consent are particularly pertinent here for example in scenarios where these medication are prescribed in the context of polypharmacy for individuals with serious mental illness or more mild forms, who push the prescribing relationship towards consumerism. Despite these challenges it is important to consider and discuss the deprescribing of these medications due to their long-term risks, including tolerance and dependence. Particular to this chapter, the prescriber may find themselves in a position of disagreement with the patient, for example—asserting a need for deprescribing in the face of a request to refill or even up-titrate. As these drugs can have varying degrees of addiction potential, we reference some strategies that are used primarily in the treatment of substance use disorders. We suggest that such strategies and interventions may be adapted when deprescribing these medications—as long as the treater remains mindful of potential harm and monitors intended outcomes. Rigorous trials are warranted to validate this approach. In this chapter we focus on the management of the medication regimen and the original indication for the prescription. We do not dwell on the co-occurring substance use disorders (when present in the case examples) as the treatment of addictions per se is beyond the scope of this book and well-covered elsewhere. Throughout this chapter, we also subscribe to a "harm-reduction" approach, now widely accepted in the treatment of addictions.

Goals and Learning Objectives

After reading this chapter, the reader will be able to:

1. Name three pharmacological management strategies for prescription benzodiazepine (BZD) dependence
2. Describe some the common reasons for deprescribing stimulants
3. Outline three strategies for deprescribing stimulants

Case Example

Jason is a 40-year-old man who has severe social anxiety disorder and alcohol use disorder. He stays home all day watching TV and drinks 5–6 beers every night. He has also taken clonazepam 1 mg three times a day for the past 7 years initiated by his now retired primary care provider. His new primary care provider is concerned about the combination of alcohol and the benzodiazepine (BZD) and suggests reducing the total daily dose by 0.5 mg. Jason loses his temper, declares he is not "an addict", and leaves the office angrily.

This is unfortunately not an uncommon scenario in clinical practice. The prescriber has the unenviable burden of a clear rationale to deprescribe the BZD due to a risk of dependence and additive effects with alcohol. The timing, however, is suboptimal. On the next visit, the prescriber suggests a consultation with a specialist (an addictions psychiatrist) who validates that the clonazepam should be eventually deprescribed but commits to preventing an abrupt withdrawal. This prescriber also manages to reflect back and validate the patient's anger and fear at this proposal as a first step. They next begin to explore the history and meaning of alcohol use for this patient.

Deprescribing Medication with Abuse Potential or Rewarding Effects: Common Challenges

This chapter combines a discussion of several medications that share common properties in terms of their risk of dependence and tendency to be misused. Rewarding effects of medications may be mediated via classic addiction pathways i.e. mu opioid receptor activation and activation of the nucleus accumbens. In general the greater rapidity of onset of effects, the greater the liability of reward. The immediate relief of an adverse emotional state (e.g. alprazolam for a panic attack) can be extremely reinforcing from a learning theory standpoint. Reduction and/or discontinuation of these medications may involve particular difficulties, including but not limited to (1) the patient being unwilling to discontinue them; (2) severe withdrawal symptoms (e.g. seizures and delirium with BZDs); (3) other withdrawal symptoms including depressive symptoms, persistent anxiety, and insomnia; and (4) an almost immediate reappearance of symptoms that the medications were initiated for (such as lack of concentration, hyperactivity, anxiety, or insomnia). These common challenges can be approached in a variety of ways, but there may be increased risk of emergence of countertransferential reactions (e.g. based on a lack of hope of recovery, or past breeches in alliance and perceived trust with former patients).

It can be challenging for prescribers to maintain a balanced therapeutic stance when consumeristic patients request or even demand specific medications with abuse potential in lieu of discussing reasonable alternatives. These dynamics can similarly present when attempting to deprescribe such medications—with the added potential of having to simultaneously manage a withdrawal syndrome. Such patients may intimidate prescribers, eliciting reactions of fear, helplessness, anger, and guilt. These scenarios can be exceptionally anxiety-provoking for trainees. A useful question to ask when either patient or prescriber proposes a prescription change is "what are the underlying reasons?" This allows the prescriber to attempt to understand the manifest and latent content of the decision-making process for the partnership. When managing potential countertransference, treaters should remain equally aware of the risk of reaction formation and seek an neutral, balanced stance. Periodically assessing where the collaboration sits on the continuum of shared decision making (from consumerism to paternalism) is a useful grounding exercise here. Emotional reactions, for example, evoked by a patient's demands to continue or titrate a counter-therapeutic medication are normal, but may also be a worthy focus of peer supervision or the prescriber's own therapy.

Similarly, identifying and processing the patient's feelings in a nonjudg-mental fashion may help maintain the relationship and prevent behaviors unconsciously motivated by negative reactions. Scratching the surface of the patient's request also helps the prescriber further develop empathy, which in turn fosters the maintenance of a therapeutic approach. The pre-scriber would do well to be aware of the power struggles and psychological reactance that may emerge when interacting with an assertive patient. In a situation where a patient demands a BZD or a stimulant, the power balance may feel tilted as each party tries to exercise its autonomy at the expense of the other. In this setting, patients may feel as if the prescriber is "holding them hostage" by deliberately refusing medications. Prescribers, in turn, may feel pressured because their medical knowledge and authority is being challenged.

Closely related to the idea of power struggles is the concept of *psycholog-ical reactance*—the tendency to deny requests out of hand as a consequence of perceived threats to autonomy. This natural human tendency can play out unnoticed in prescribing relationships. As mentioned in Chapter 3, the theory of psychological reactance states that individuals have certain free-doms with regard to their behavior which, when curtailed or threatened will lead to the individual being motivationally aroused to regain them (see Brehm, 1966). An example of psychological reactance would be a situation where a patient comes into the office requesting a prescription for alpra-zolam during a deprescribing effort of clonazepam. The prescriber may have an immediate reaction such as, "I am the prescriber here and I decide on which medication, when and how much. Why are you telling me how to do my job?". This may be an uncomfortable reaction to acknowledge be-cause it is counter to the perceived identity of healer and empathic provider. But in acknowledging this response (which is not to be judged but instead considered as part of the range of human experience in such a scenario) the prescriber can question their own reaction and potentially utilize it as data about the relationship with the patient.

When there is clear and persistent disagreement regarding a course of action, getting a second opinion from another provider may be an option. Shared decision making does not mean that the prescriber will not be held responsible for unsafe prescriptions, and it is completely acceptable—and indeed, expected—that the prescriber will refuse to participate in a plan that is unsafe.

Deprescribing Benzodiazepines

BZD and related drugs (z-drugs) are widely used to treat anxiety disorders and insomnia. It has been established that they can cause tolerance and physiological and psychological dependence as well as serious side effects and interactions with alcohol and other medications (such as opioids). Some recommendations advise they be prescribed only for short periods of time (e.g. up to 2–4 weeks, see Ashton, 2005) due to a risk of dependence (Murphy & Tyrer, 1991), but, in real-world practice, these drugs are often continued for much longer periods of time.

Long-term use of these medications can have negative effects beyond addiction and dependence formation. For example the long-term use of BZDs into older adulthood has been shown to be associated with a higher risk of cognitive decline and dementia (see de Gage et al., 2012; Pariente, de Gage, Moore, & Bégaud, 2016). The overuse and abuse of prescription BZDs has received increased public health focus more recently, being considered by some as the next wave of the 'opioid epidemic'. At the same time, these medications have largely unrivaled utility in the immediate management of anxiety, making the dilemma of prescribing and deprescribing more challenging. Although numerous studies can be found to guide deprescribing BZDs in older adults in either primary care or nursing homes (thanks to the field of geriatrics), almost no literature exists in more general psychiatric populations.

Potential Indications for Deprescribing BDZs

The recommendation for time-limited use means the initial prescription of a BZD in itself demands an expectation and plan in place for deprescribing them. There are however other situations where it may be necessary to help the patient discontinue. Examples include additive or interactive effects of problem alcohol use, or coincident use of prescription opioids such as methadone maintenance treatment—both of which significantly increase the risk of respiratory depression and death (see McCance-Katz, Sullivan, & Nallani, 2010; Tanaka, 2002). BZDs may interact with antihypertensive, antipsychotic, and certain oral hypoglycemic agents for example, to increase the risk of falls in elderly individuals. Although it may be appropriate to preemptively deprescribe BZDs to *avoid* the development of dependence and abuse, the appearance of any sign of dependence (see Box 11.1) makes the discussion more urgent. On some occasions, patient may themselves initiate the discussion about deprescribing BZDs out of related concerns. Prescribers should also consider the potential construct of 'pseudoaddiction' where apparent 'medication seeking' and behavioral signs of addiction are a manifestation of undertreatment of the underlying condition (such as an anxiety disorder).

Box 11.1 Possible Features of BDZ Dose Dependence

- Patient has taken benzodiazepenes (BZDs) in prescribed (usually low) doses for months or years.
- Patient has gradually begun to "need" BZDs to carry out normal, day-to-day activities.
- Patient has continued to take BZD although the original indication for prescription has disappeared.
- Patient has difficulty in stopping the drug, or reducing dosage, because of withdrawal symptoms.
- If on short-acting BZDs, they develop anxiety symptoms between doses or get a craving for the next dose.
- Patient contacts their prescriber regularly to obtain repeat prescriptions and become anxious if the next prescription is not readily available.
- Patient may have increased the dosage since the original prescription.
- Patient may have anxiety symptoms, panics, agoraphobia, insomnia, depression, and increasing physical symptoms despite continuing to take BZDs.

From the "Ashton Manual," C. H. Ashton (2002).

The approach to deprescribing BZDs will depend on whether the patient (1) is using prescribed doses or overusing; (2) demonstrating features of dependence such as craving, tolerance, withdrawal (3) demonstrating features of comorbid addiction such as drug-seeking, alternative sources, detrimental functional impact related to use; or (4) is invested in deprescribing and using non-BZD strategies to manage withdrawal. To gain a patient perspective, a qualitative study worthy of further reading, analyzed internet forum discussions of former-BZD users and framed seven themes in the process of recovery from BZD use: "hell and isolation, anxiety and depression, alienation, physical distress, anger and remorse, waves and windows, and healing and renewal" (see Fixsen & Ridge, 2017).

Pharmacological Strategies

Tapering Schedules

Most guidelines for BZD discontinuation recommend a taper, the duration of which may range from a few weeks to a year (see Ashton, 2005). Reminiscent of antidepressants, online forums of former-BZD users mention strategies such as "micro-tapering," which may involve tapering doses by as little as 5–10% a month. These forums also use terminology such as "dry tapers" (referring to the pills being cut or crushed using a pill-cutter) or "wet tapers" where the pills are dissolved in commercially available water-based vehicles to dissolve them such as "OraPlus." In the context of established diagnosable longterm benzodiazepine dependence longer tapers (last months) are indicated.

Treating Withdrawal Symptoms

BZDs can cause serious and life-threatening withdrawal symptoms including catatonia, psychosis, delirium, and seizures (see Mackinnon & Parker, 1982; Schweizer & Rickels, 1998) in addition to intense short-term anxiety and insomnia. Similar withdrawal symptoms have been reported with zolpidem (Victorri-Vigneau et al., 2014) and zopiclone (Flynn & Cox, 2006). A protracted BZD withdrawal syndrome that is proposed by some

Table 11.1 Examples of Commonly prescribed benzodiazepines, z-drugs, and stimulants

Medication class	Common medications
Benzodiazepines	Alprazolam, clonazepam, lorazepam, diazepam
Z-drugs	Zolpidem, zopiclone, eszopiclone, zaleplon
Stimulants	Methylphenidate, mixed amphetamine salts, lisdexamphetamine, dexamphetamine

and reported in up to 10–15% patients is less well-known and studied (see Ashton, 1995; Higgitt, Fonagy, Toone, & Shine, 1990). This syndrome is purported to last from months to years and is characterized by persistent anxiety and insomnia due to receptor adaptation, as well as psychological difficulties (such as poor coping).

Distressing withdrawal symptoms have been cited as the main reason for relapse to the use of BZDs or an inability to stop using prescription BZDs; hence, the treatment of withdrawal symptoms is critical to deprescribing BZDs. The first approach is typically tapering with medications within the same class—typically those BDZs with longer half lifes such as clonazepam or diazepam. More rapid BDZ self taper protocols do exist *for the acute treatment of alcohol withdrawal* (e.g. with chlordiazepoxide) in ER or IP settings. However, without appropriate provision for continuing multi-dimensional care this arguably reflects a suboptimal approach. Anticonvulsants such as carbamazepine (Denis, Fatseas, Lavie, & Auriacombe, 2006) and pregabalin (Bobes et al., 2012) have been used to replace BDZs when managing withdrawal. However, caution is advised with the use of pregabalin and gabapentin because they can themselves cause dependence (see Schifano, 2014).

Less acute withdrawal symptoms such as insomnia may be management with alternative hypnotics (such as low dose trazodone, over the counter sleep aids or melatonin). Anxiety may warrant the use of as needed hydroxyzine or propranolol or a standing SSRI. Given the broad tranquilizing effects of BDZs, during deprescribng, prescribers should remain vigilant to the possibility of uncovering a previously unrecognized psychiatric disorder (such as a mood diathesis or even psychosis), previously masked by the BDZ. In these scenarios more targeted pharmacotherapy may be necessary.

Psychotherapeutic Interventions

Cognitive behavior therapy for the management of insomnia (CBT-I) and for anxiety, when initiated before a BZD taper may ease the distress from BZD withdrawal. Both these interventions have been discussed in greater detail in Chapter 6. In addition to individual therapy, groups and communities of former-users can prove to be valuable supports during BZD deprescribing.

Community Strategies, Population-Based Interventions and Education

In community-dwelling older adults direct-to-consumer educational interventions such as "EMPOWER" have been shown to stimulate conversation and shared decision-making around the use of BZDs (see Tannenbaum, Martin, Tamblyn, Benedetti, & Ahmed, 2014). Public education through advertising campaigns, community forums, and reading materials about the dangers of long-term BZD use are warranted to reduce the risk that this class follows the same path as prescription opiates in their association with the opioid epidemic—a current public health crisis across the US and beyond.

Deprescribing Stimulant Medications

Deprescribing stimulants can be challenging because some effects are desirable and can in fact be harnessed to enhance performance in the short term, rather than address a deficit (see Bossaer et al., 2013). Stimulants are an evidenced based and life-changing treatment when prescriber appropriately for the management of ADHD, ADD and some subtypes of depression. Therefore their therapeutic use should not carry stigma. Given comorbid substance use disorders are an important factor when considering and planning any deprescribing, treaters should remain mindful of the high rates of addiction reported in patients with ADHD. Comorbid ADHD and substance use disorder is not considered an absolute contraindication to prescribing stimulants.

Unfortunately, some reasons why stimulant medications are desirable to some individuals for non-clinical use include:

- Immediate-release formulations produce a euphoric effect and an increase in energy and alertness.
- Oral preparations can be modified for more rapid onset (e.g. ground and snorted).
- They can be sold for money or bartered for other drugs, alcohol, or sex.
- Patients may have had prior experiences with them as pediatricians, primary care physicians, and psychiatrists prescribe them therefore they are prevalent, commonly diverted and perceived to be safe.
- They can improve performance at work or academics in a relatively short time.

As child psychiatry is beyond of the scope of this book, we will be discussing deprescribing of stimulants only among adult patients. Stimulant medications are used for the treatment of ADHD in both children and adults. A study on stimulant prescription patterns from 2006 to 2009 showed that the number of prescriptions increased by 34% each year, with a disproportionate increase among women and adults (Zetterqvist, Asherson, Halldner, Långström, & Larsson, 2013). In addition to ADHD, stimulants may be prescribed for treatment-resistant depression (Stotz, Woggon, & Angst, 1999), in post-stroke depression to enhance participation in physical therapy (Grade, Redford, Chrostowski, Toussaint, & Blackwell, 1998), as augmentation in geriatric depression (Lavretsky, Park, Siddarth, Kumar, & Reynolds III, 2006; Lavretsky et al., 2015), and medically in patients for a variety of reasons (Masand & Tesar, 1996). As with other classes of psychotropic medications, guidelines are provided for the initiation and continuation of stimulants, regrettably (with the exception of temporary 'drug holidays' in ADHD treatment) with relatively little information on how or when to discontinue them.

Potential Indications for Deprescribing Stimulants

Stimulants can have serious side effects such as increasing heart rate and blood pressure, cardiac events, loss of appetite and weight, tics, obsessive-compulsive behavior, psychotic symptoms, and mania. Although side effects may be managed through dose adjustment or by the addition of another medication (such as a mood stabilizer or an antipsychotic medication) some situations may warrant discontinuation of the stimulant itself.

As covered above with BZDs, if a patient shows signs of developing misuse/dependence efforts should be made to prevent or manage this comorbidity. Furthermore, if prescribed medications are being distributed or sold ("diversion") or snorted, crushed, and injected intravenously, these are strong grounds for discontinuation.

When stimulants are prescribed for short-term indications, such as for improvement of participation in physical therapy following a stroke or for augmentation of Alzheimer's disease treatment, plans and expectations for deprescribing should be established at time of initial prescribing.

Stimulant Withdrawal Symptoms

There is a vastly greater literature describing withdrawal syndromes related to stimulant abuse than to clinical use, suggesting that the former syndrome is more common and significant. Although generally not considered life threatening (as compared to BDZ withdrawal), severe psychological discomfort is reported during withdrawal from stimulant (i.e. amphetamine) abuse and can escalate to include dangerous agitation or severe depression with suicidality. Commonly reported symptoms include: dysphoria, fatigue, insomnia, hypersomnia, psychomotor agitation, increased appetite, unpleasant dreams, irritability, aches and pain and social withdrawal.

In terms of withdrawal from appropriate clinical use, two case reports, both in children, have described the appearance of depressive symptoms—with psychotic features in one case—following the withdrawal of stimulant medication (methylphenidate and pemoline; see Brown, Borden, Spunt, & Medenis, 1985; Rosenfeld, 1979). One case report describes the appearance of dystonia during withdrawal in a man who had used up to 600 mg/d of methylphenidate (Grau-López, Daigre, Mercado, Casas, & Roncero, 2017).

A small study of abrupt stimulant withdrawal in children with comorbid ADHD and tic disorder showed that there was no worsening of tics, but the children who continued to take the stimulants did better on measures of ADHD. The authors concluded that abrupt stimulant withdrawal was not deleterious but that this "did not preclude the development of withdrawal reactions in susceptible individuals" (Nolan, Gadow, & Sprafkin, 1999).

Pharmacological Strategies for Managing Deprescribing of Stimulants

A 'stimulant holiday' is a construct apparently more established in child than adult psychiatry, where, for example a child's ADHD medication is temporary suspended over the weekend or school break when symptoms may be less problematic. Generally, tapers are not recommended. Withdrawal syndromes from prescription doses of stimulants have not been heavily features in formal medical literature and there are no established pharmacological strategies for management. Two randomized controlled trials have shown the utility of bupropion in the treatment of mild methamphetamine *dependence* in conjunction with behavior therapy (see Elkashef et al., 2008; Shoptaw et al., 2008). In adults who have used prescription stimulants such as mixed amphetamine salts for long periods of time with signs of dependence (and risk of major depression), it might be reasonable to trial bupropion in the peri-deprescribing period. Bupropion offers the other potential benefits of treating emergent depression or recurrence of attentional deficits.

Conclusion

BZDs and stimulant medications may be priorities for deprescribing from the prescriber's point of view due to concerns about diversion, dependence and abuse; however they may be very desirable to the patient. Due to these conflicts, it may be especially important to educate the patient about side effects and maintain a strong alliance while also maintaining clear boundaries around safety. BZDs may have a prolonged and distressing withdrawal syndrome that can be life-threatening in the acute stages, thus necessitating a very slow taper that can run into years. Although stimulant withdrawal syndromes are not well documented in literature, case reports indicate that depressive syndromes can develop during the withdrawal which may warrant treatment.

Case Examples

Case Example 1

Jen, a 43-year-old woman, was prescribed citalopram and clonazepam to treat a generalized anxiety disorder that emerged following a divorce. Her anxiety symptoms and sleep improved instantly, and she continued to go about her daily routine. After 8 weeks, her prescriber suggested discontinuing the clonazepam because of the risk of dependence. Jen agreed, and the medication was tapered over 4 weeks. Jen remained asymptomatic until the dose was reduced to 0.5 mg twice a day. Any dose below that produced severe anxiety. Eight weeks later, the dose was increased again to 1 mg twice a day by a covering physician. When Jen was approached about reducing clonazepam a year later, she seemed very conflicted because she recalled the side effects she had experienced and also feared withdrawal seizures (see Tables 11.1 and 11.2).

Table 11.2 Decision making grid for case 1

Decision-making grid		
	Risks	Benefits
Continuing clonazepam	Long-term side effects including dependence, memory loss, risk of falls, drug interactions	Treatment of withdrawal symptoms
Deprescribing clonazepam	Withdrawal symptoms Time and labor-intensive process	Development of non-pharmacological strategies

Patient values/preference: Patient prefers to continue clonazepam because the last experience of withdrawal was very distressing. At the same time, the patient understands the risks of long term BZD use and wants to stop using them.

Plan: Deprescribe clonazepam

Interventions: Start psychotherapy for anxiety and insomnia before changing the dose of clonazepam, emphasize that the plan is flexible, keep the rate of taper slow, allow for extended periods on the same dose if needed, delay the taper if there are stressors that the patient finds distressing, discuss the possibility of small as-needed doses for "bad" days.

Case Example 2

Joe is a 56-year-old man with a history of cocaine dependence after which he developed a generalized anxiety disorder. He also has hypertension, diabetes, and hepatitis C. He takes fluoxetine and clonazepam 1 mg three times a day. Every time his prescriber suggests reducing the BZD, he says that he cannot go through withdrawal and that he would die without taking BZDs (see Table 11.3).

Table 11.3 Decision making grid for case 2

Decision-making grid	Risks	Benefits
Continuing clonazepam	Long-term side effects	It is what the patient wants; no clinical benefit
Deprescribing clonazepam	Withdrawal symptoms Time and labor-intensive process	Development of non-pharmacological strategies

Patient values/preference: Patient does not want any change in the dose of clonazepam

Plan: Continue psychoeducation

Interventions: Psychoeducation, CBT for anxiety symptoms

Case Example 3

Dan is a 55-year-old man with severe depression and posttraumatic stress disorder (PTSD). He was prescribed methylphenidate in addition to an SSRI on an inpatient service where he was admitted for suicidality. He states that it really helps him get through the day and is asking you to increase the dose by 5 mg twice a day. He is unwilling to discuss any reduction in the dose. When informed about side effects he says "My life is terrible already. I don't care about a few side effects if it helps me get through the day." See Table 11.4.

Table 11.4 Decision making grid for case 3

Decision-making grid

	Risks	Benefits
Continuing methylphenidate	Long-term side effects, risk of dependence	It is what the patient wants; no clinical benefit
Deprescribing methylphenidate	Patient will drop out of treatment	Development of non-pharmacological strategies

Patient values/preference: Patient wants an increase in the dose

Plan: Continue psychoeducation

Self-Assessment

1. Tom has been taking clonazepam 3 mg total daily for the past 7 years. He came across an article in the newspaper that said that he could develop dementia. He is terrified, abruptly stopped taking the clonazepam, and has a panic attack. Now he refuses to "touch the stuff."

   a. What is your initial intervention with Tom?

   b. What will you suggest as a long-term plan?

2. Tina was given methylphenidate by her roommate as a trial. She liked the effect and had her doctor prescribe it monthly for the next 6 months. She now says that she finds it impossible to even make her bed if she doesn't take it.

   a. What do you think is the cause of Tina's complaint?

   b. What will you suggest to Tina?

References

Ashton, H. (1995). Protracted withdrawal from benzodiazepines: The post-withdrawal syndrome. *Psychiatric Annals*, 25(3), 174–179.

Ashton, H. (2005). The diagnosis and management of benzodiazepine dependence. *Current Opinion in Psychiatry, 18*(3), 249–255.

Bossaer, J. B., Gray, J. A., Miller, S. E., Enck, G., Gaddipati, V. C., & Enck, R. E. (2013). The use and misuse of prescription stimulants as "cognitive enhancers" by students at one academic health sciences center. *Academic Medicine, 88*(7), 967–971.

Brehm, J. W. (1966). *A theory of psychological reactance.* Oxford, England: Academic Press.

Brown, R., Borden, K., Spunt, A., & Medenis, R. (1985). Depression following pemoline withdrawal in a hyperactive child. *Clinical Pediatrics, 24*(3), 174.

de Gage, S. B., Bégaud, B., Bazin, F., Verdoux, H., Dartigues, J.-F., Pérès, K., . . . Pariente, A. (2012). Benzodiazepine use and risk of dementia: Prospective population based study. *British Medical Journal, 345*, e6231.

Denis, C., Fatseas, M., Lavie, E., & Auriacombe, M. (2006). Pharmacological interventions for benzodiazepine mono-dependence management in outpatient settings. *Cochrane Database of Systematic Reviews,* (3).

Elkashef, A. M., Rawson, R. A., Anderson, A. L., Li, S.-H., Holmes, T., Smith, E. V., . . . Ling, W. (2008). Bupropion for the treatment of methamphetamine dependence. *Neuropsychopharmacology, 33*(5), 1162.

Fixsen, A. M., & Ridge, D. (2017). Stories of hell and healing: Internet users' construction of benzodiazepine distress and withdrawal. *Qualitative Health Research, 27*(13), 2030–2041.

Flynn, A., & Cox, D. (2006). Dependence on zopiclone. *Addiction, 101*(6), 898.

Grade, C., Redford, B., Chrostowski, J., Toussaint, L., & Blackwell, B. (1998). Methylphenidate in early poststroke recovery: A double-blind, placebo-controlled study. *Archives of Physical Medicine and Rehabilitation, 79*(9), 1047–1050.

Grau-López, L., Daigre, C., Mercado, N., Casas, M., & Roncero, C. (2017). Dystonia in methylphenidate withdrawal: A case report. *Journal of Addiction Medicine, 11*(2), 154–156.

Higgitt, A., Fonagy, P., Toone, B., & Shine, P. (1990). The prolonged benzodiazepine withdrawal syndrome: Anxiety or hysteria? *Acta Psychiatrica Scandinavica, 82*(2), 165–168.

Lavretsky, H., Park, S., Siddarth, P., Kumar, A., & Reynolds III, C. F. (2006). Methylphenidate-enhanced antidepressant response to citalopram in the elderly: A double-blind, placebo-controlled pilot trial. *American Journal of Geriatric Psychiatry, 14*(2), 181–185.

Lavretsky, H., Reinlieb, M., St. Cyr, N., Siddarth, P., Ercoli, L. M., & Senturk, D. (2015). Citalopram, methylphenidate, or their combination in geriatric depression: A randomized, double-blind, placebo-controlled trial. *American Journal of Psychiatry, 172*(6), 561–569.

Mackinnon, G. L., & Parker, W. A. (1982). Benzodiazepine withdrawal syndrome: A literature review and evaluation. *American Journal of Drug and Alcohol Abuse, 9*(1), 19–33.

Masand, P. S., & Tesar, G. E. (1996). Use of stimulants in the medically ill. *Psychiatric Clinics of North America, 19*(3), 515–547.

McCance-Katz, E. F., Sullivan, L. E., & Nallani, S. (2010). Drug interactions of clinical importance among the opioids, methadone and buprenorphine, and other frequently prescribed medications: A review. *American Journal on Addictions, 19*(1), 4–16.

Murphy, S. M., & Tyrer, P. (1991). A double-blind comparison of the effects of gradual withdrawal of lorazepam, diazepam and bromazepam in benzodiazepine dependence. *British Journal of Psychiatry, 158*(4), 511–516.

Nolan, E. E., Gadow, K. D., & Sprafkin, J. (1999). Stimulant medication withdrawal during long-term therapy in children with comorbid attention-deficit hyperactivity disorder and chronic multiple tic disorder. *Pediatrics, 103*(4), 730–737.

Pariente, A., de Gage, S. B., Moore, N., & Bégaud, B. (2016). The benzodiazepine–dementia disorders link: Current state of knowledge. *CNS Drugs, 30*(1), 1–7.

Rosenfeld, A. A. (1979). Depression and psychotic regression following prolonged methylphenidate use and withdrawal: Case report. *American Journal of Psychiatry, 136*(2), 226–228.

Schifano, F. (2014). Misuse and abuse of pregabalin and gabapentin: cause for concern? *CNS Drugs, 28*(6), 491–496.

Schweizer, E., & Rickels, K. (1998). Benzodiazepine dependence and withdrawal: A review of the syndrome and its clinical management. *Acta Psychiatrica Scandinavica, 98*(s393), 95–101.

Shoptaw, S., Heinzerling, K. G., Rotheram-Fuller, E., Steward, T., Wang, J., Swanson, A.-N., . . . Ling, W. (2008). Randomized, placebo-controlled trial of bupropion for the treatment of methamphetamine dependence. *Drug and Alcohol Dependence, 96*(3), 222–232.

Stotz, G., Woggon, B., & Angst, J. (1999). Psychostimulants in the therapy of treatment-resistant depression: Review of the literature and findings from a retrospective study in 65 depressed patients. *Dialogues in Clinical Neuroscience, 1*(3), 165.

Tanaka, E. (2002). Toxicological interactions between alcohol and benzodiazepines. *Journal of Toxicology: Clinical Toxicology, 40*(1), 69–75.

Tannenbaum, C., Martin, P., Tamblyn, R., Benedetti, A., & Ahmed, S. (2014). Reduction of inappropriate benzodiazepine prescriptions among older adults through direct patient education: The EMPOWER cluster randomized trial. *JAMA Internal Medicine, 174*(6), 890–898.

Victorri-Vigneau, C., Gerardin, M., Rousselet, M., Guerlais, M., Grall-Bronnec, M., & Jolliet, P. (2014). An update on zolpidem abuse and dependence. *Journal of Addictive Diseases, 33*(1), 15–23.

Zetterqvist, J., Asherson, P., Halldner, L., Långström, N., & Larsson, H. (2013). Stimulant and non-stimulant attention deficit/hyperactivity disorder drug use: Total population study of trends and discontinuation patterns 2006–2009. *Acta Psychiatrica Scandinavica, 128*(1), 70–77.

12

Concluding Thoughts and
Future Directions

In this concluding chapter, we summarize the major points of the book and identify future directions for research and practice in the topic of deprescribing.

What We Hope You Take Away from This Book

Over the past few years of putting this book together, the landscape around the topic of deprescribing in psychiatry has begun to significantly shift and expand. More focus on the concerns of long-term psychotropic drug use has been emerging in the literature as well as in the popular press. This is evidenced by numerous publications and articles about antidepressant withdrawal symptoms (Davies & Read, 2018; Read, Cartwright, & Gibson, 2018), the emerging epidemic of benzodiazepine addiction (Weaver, 2018), with its similarities to the opioid crisis, and greater recognition of the lay literature and online forums which address discontinuing psychiatric medications. On the other hand, the mainstream literature has provided further evidence *for* rational polypharmacy and *against* safe AP discontinuation in schizophrenia. Even mortality as an outcome may be of relative value to those favoring quality of life. Interpretation of this literature appears to be largely dependent on the outcomes most commonly used in these studies (hospitalization rates, positive symptoms severity, functional recovery, or cardiovascular risk) and the usual inferential limitations of large observational studies. Patient forums offering support and anecdotal guidance on self-tapering strategies (e.g. minute dosing via oral suspensions) are gaining traction but are mostly unfrequented or unknown by treaters. If psychiatry does not earn a seat at the table when critical decisions are being made by our patients, an opportunity is missed. This brings us to our first "take home" from this book: Do ask, do tell.

Do Ask, Do Tell

Your patients may already be doing "DIY deprescribing," and you, as the prescriber, may not know unless you bring up the topic. If your patients express any interest in reducing or stopping their medications, it is possible that some have already started the process if not already stopped medications completely. Seize the opportunity to start this conversation, and do not take lightly their broaching of the topic. The power differential between prescriber and patient should not be underestimated and can manifest as fear of expressing the desire to reduce or stop a medication you are prescribing.

Further, one might bookmark the option of an eventual collaborative discontinuation—at the time of initiation of a medication—interleaving deprescribing with prescribing as two sides of the same coin. When initiating a medication, one should actively discuss with the patient both their expectations of how long the medication will be taken as well as your own thoughts and recommendations. Our stance is that psychiatry as a field must question the assumption and temper the implication that medications, when initiated, should be continued indefinitely. We suggest considering deprescribing as potentially as viable an intervention as prescribing when appropriate. New evidence can and will emerge on the level of individual patient, and without adequate expertise in deprescribing we will not be prepared to respond. Even the paradigm of insulin management of diabetes (so often borrowed to evoke the rationale for life-long psychopharmacotherapy) is called into question both as the metaphor of a chemical imbalance explaining mental illness is reconsidered, and as deprescribing of insulin is being considered for some established cases of diabetes mellitus. Similarly, the risk/benefit ratio guiding the (previously well accepted) recommendation of low dose aspirin for secondary prevention of cardiovascular disease has recently shifted.

Along with introducing the deprescribing process at the initiation of a new medication, it is also essential to remain open to discussing the possibility of decreasing or discontinuing those medications the person is currently taking (even if contrary to your recommendation). One certainly has the responsibility of raising the issue if there are clear and significant risks of continuing the current regimen even if the patient may not be interested in decreasing medications. A periodic, collaborative review of the medication list, along with a clear description of the current risks and benefits to continuing the regimen, is important to demonstrate interest in our patient's and judiousness in our prescribing. Accepting these discussions may not result in a change, but as circumstances change, new evidence emerges and the therapeutic alliance deepens, opportunities to deprescribe may present themselves.

It's the Relationship

Working together in a collaborative fashion is key in all of medicine but particularly in psychiatry. Keeping in mind the multiple and potentially conflicting meanings of the prescription is essential to the process. Creating an atmosphere where deprescribing can be done together, in a way that considers the expertise and experience of both prescriber and patient, can develop a space where issues that were not previously raised may emerge in the process of discussing medications. Shared decision-making often involves shared risk-taking—an endeavor which, if done right, can forge a strong therapeutic alliance.

Alongside the therapeutic relationship with the prescriber, examining a patient's whole constellation of relationships is important. Problematic relationships in a patient's life might have gone unrecognized or unaddressed by virtue of collateral effects of the now discontinued medication. The role of "identified patient" within a family or social system may start to shift as deprescribing is implemented; how this impacts the family constellation and the ripple effects it causes may have more dramatic effects than anticipated.

Finally, the patient's relationship to the medication, the treatment, and, ultimately, to him- or herself as a person taking or not taking medications can cause other shifts. Identity around being a "patient" or inhabiting the "sick role" may start to change. Complex feelings may emerge. There may be grief as well as joy: joy for those who have waited a long time to stop medications and are happy with the results; and grief at not having tried this sooner. There may be strong feelings toward former (or current) treaters, related to the initial prescribing. All of these relationships and emerging emotions are ripe areas for addressing and potential areas for growth.

Be Prepared

Planning ahead with the patient is another area of focus in pursuing deprescribing. Preparing the ground for the successful trial of a reduction or discontinuation of medications requires thoughtfulness and additional work, but it is an investment that stands to pay off in the future.

Planning how to pursue deprescribing includes working to prepare a comprehensive medication list that includes intended/anticipated benefits and risks for the prescription of each. Identifying which medications would be the top candidates to start the medication reduction can be helpful especially if the patient is interested but unsure of where to start. Part of preparing for deprescribing also includes potentially protecting extra time to check in on how the patient is doing, particularly in the beginning days and weeks of this effort.

Preparing for reactions and discomfort from other people in the patient's life is important. For example, the visiting nurse who oversees medication administration may be taken aback by the idea that the prescriber is reducing the use of an antipsychotic medication (without the introduction of another in its place). The family, who may have experience-based fears around the patient not taking medication, can be very distressed when they find out about this course of action if they are not prepared and on board with the decision.

Preparation extends to creating a wellness plan with the patient or encouraging them to do so on their own. Chapters 5 and 6 reviewed different types of preplanning tools to support the patient in reflecting on past experiences of increased distress and in identifying specific plans in the event that the patient needs to be hospitalized. Putting these in place prior to pursuing any reduction of medications can offer the patient and the prescriber, as well as others involved, an increased sense of comfort and control. A patient may choose not to share these plans with others or may only share with providers; this is a personal choice to be respected. Finding a format, tone, and approach that feels culturally and personally relevant is important with these plans; one size does not fit all in this very personal of processes.

Prepare the person (and their support system/treatment team) for a potential increase in feelings—feelings they may have avoided or that may have been dulled by the sedating effects of the medication. The recognition and management of these feelings is an important area of focus because the emergence of strong feelings may be mistaken for a return of symptoms, especially in the case of long-term overmedication.

"First You Leap, Then You Grow Wings"

This quote, by the theologian William Sloan Coffin (2004), illustrates the importance of allowing a "good enough" starting point for deprescribing in psychiatry, ahead of and as we build the necessary evidence base to support more definitive and specific clinical guidelines. The construct of clinical practice guiding research is readily accepted (and has proved quite successful), as in the off-label use of medications. "Off-label" prescribing (and deprescribing) must be practiced with due diligence, the full informed consent of the patient, and in good faith. The individual sitting in front of you in your office may be suffering or, even more insidiously, surviving but not actually thriving. In a bid to be cautious and adhere purely to empirically supported treatments (e.g., where meta-analyses or consensus guidelines exist), we may miss the evidence sitting in front of us. We should not forget that "evidence-based practice" must include clinical judgment and patient preferences in equal partnership with the evidence-based treatments. Coffin (2004), encourages us: "One must, in short, dare to act wholeheartedly without absolute certainty". The mandate of the complex conditions within which we treat is that we cannot let the perfect be the enemy of the good, and at times we must act without the luxury of certain evidence.

In the same way that we must have courage in pursing changes in treatment, we need to encourage our patients to try, to risk, to take chances, to *live*. Deprescribing is certainly not the only avenue to this, but to harken back to the prologue of the book where we quoted Deegan (2004) and the experience of "what it means to be buried under an avalanche of psychiatric drugs" for a number of the patients with whom we work, this may in fact the status quo with which we collude. Symptoms may be reduced, but at a cost to the person's feeling of being alive or fully participating in their life.

To reiterate the position as laid out in this book: psychiatric medications have proved useful and beneficial, and many, many people would attribute much of their current fulfilling lives to the assistance and existence of these drugs. But those (often vulnerable) individuals who are 'buried' should be granted the opportunity to try digging themselves out. To support and assist with the collaborative inquiry that is deprescribing requires rigor, ethics, courage, and the wide support of the field and systems in which we practice.

A Call for Research

The research base for deprescribing in psychiatry is in its infancy but can leverage (with caveats) experimental and observation studies published on medication discontinuation. While we can draw from other fields of medicine and guidelines developed around (specifically) decreasing polypharmacy in those specialties, we have argued here that psychiatry presents a unique set of challenges and is not, in fact, "an illness like any other." In being an illness that is stigmatized, feared, widespread, without clear etiology, and with huge societal ramifications, the pursuit of something like deprescribing cannot be just a cookbook of guidelines and recommendations, but also requires considering the sociopolitical implications that are highlighted in policy debates, differences of opinion among advocacy groups, and promulgated each time a mass shooting is blamed on the "mental illness" of the perpetrator.

With these considerations, though, we believe strongly that a rigorous scientific investigation of deprescribing is a priority. With some initial studies showing positive indications (cf. Ostrow, Jessel, Hurd, Darrow & Cohen, 2017; Steingard, 2018), there is yet much work to be done in process research, guidelines development, outcomes research, and cost-effectiveness research.

Barriers to deprescribing have been identified here and are clear from initial studies, but these need to be further examined and elucidated. Along with identifying barriers for prescribers, we must look at possible user-friendly tools (i.e., checklists and worksheets) to support deprescribing. Tools development to help educate patients on the front end about the possibility of reducing or stopping medications (in particular for more vulnerable populations) should be readily available for prescribers to use at the point of first prescription. These kinds of decision support tools might be developed in conjunction with existing technologies such as Deegan's computer-based support tool, accessible directly prior to meeting with a provider (recoverylibrary.com). As stated, it is with humility rather than hubris that we consider this text in its first edition. We hope that our call to action falls on sympathetic, motivated, and courageous ears; contributing neither to a fad nor a "swing of the pendulum," but rather to a meaningful expansion of our field.

Future Directions in Research

- *Trials of medication withdrawal*: As we have indicated throughout this book, clinical trials of medication withdrawal are few and have significant limitations. Ideally, every time a new medication is approved by the US Food and Drug Administration (FDA), indications and method of deprescribing or discontinuation could be made a requirement for the approval. In the absence of this, studies that have a crossover design should be required to collect and analyze data regarding withdrawal symptoms during the washout from a new drug. Furthermore, trials of more complex withdrawal interventions in which the tapers are individualized and supported by the addition of individualized nonpharmacological interventions need to be conducted.
- *Qualitative studies*: Qualitative data from individual experiences of medication withdrawal can help inform potential areas of further research in the field. Themes that emerge from narrative accounts of individual medication withdrawal stories can then be further studied with quantitative methodologies. Furthermore, interventions that were found to be anecdotally useful during withdrawal may be subjected to clinical trials.
- *Receptor neuroimaging*: Although neuroreceptor changes during medication administration have been well-studied, fewer studies examine receptor changes during medication withdrawal. These would be particularly significant to elucidate the mechanisms of how withdrawal or rebound symptoms are produced and how they may be treated effectively. Such studies also may (or may not) verify the validity of syndromes, such as dopamine supersensitivity psychoses, that have only been described clinically so far. Finally, neuroimaging may provide a way to distinguish between withdrawal symptoms and relapse of the original underlying illness (for instance, for psychosis, changes in dopamine transport and uptake versus changes in receptor density and sensitivity) thereby preventing premature resumption of the psychotropic during deprescribing.

- *Pharmacoeconomics and long-term mortality/morbidity data*: In addition to clinical trials, it is important to study and demonstrate the economic benefits of deprescribing. Large databases such as Medicaid and Medicare and all payers claims databases may be tracked to determine if deprescribing is eventually cost-effective. We should remain mindful that cost-effectiveness may not be demonstrable in the short term as the immediate effect of deprescribing could involve more psychosocial treatment costs or even emergency room visits and hospitalizations. This work will hinge on multi-stakeholder agreement on meaning outcome measures and definitions of 'cost-effectiveness' and 'value' in healthcare.
- *Consumer research, informal sources, and online forums*: At this time, patients who have self-discontinued medications are an untapped resource of information about symptoms and the management of medication withdrawal. It is becoming increasingly important to develop a methodology to formally analyze and interpret the large amounts of qualitative data that are available in the form of consumer forums and chat rooms. One good example is the work of Stockman et al. (2018) which despite methodological limitations, provides a window into antidepressant withdrawal chat rooms.

Future Directions in Clinical Practice

- *Integration into behavioral health homes*: Behavioral health homes, located within mental health facilities, provide coordination of medical services for individuals with serious mental illnesses (Alexander & Druss, 2012). As their primary function is coordination and collection of medical information from various providers, they can form an excellent hub for the development and disbursement of deprescribing recommendations for a given patient.
- *Integration into electronic records and practice management reminders*: Integration of deprescribing prompts and resources into electronic medical records may encourage providers to use this intervention by influencing culture of practice and empowering providers.
- *Development of clinical tools and algorithms*: The Beers criteria were developed to help geriatricians determine the priorities for deprescribing within a given medication list. Within psychiatry, medications such as

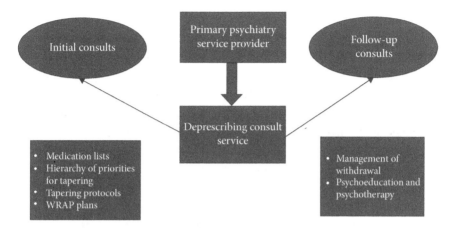

Figure 12.1 Model for a deprescribing consult service.

anticholinergics, antihistamines, and adjunctive agents could be possibly deprescribed without destabilizing the patient—it is important for us to develop similar tools. Gawande (2009) proposes that simple tools such as checklists can have powerful clinical utility.

- *Deprescribing clinics*: The formation of specialized deprescribing clinics that are focused on tracking and managing withdrawal symptoms and providing peer support, group therapy, and other nonpharmacological interventions is an important future direction.
- *Deprescribing consultation services*: Specialized consultation services on deprescribing (Figure 12.1) within a larger mental health service or using teleconferencing based consultation (such as the ECHO project) may be useful to initiate the process as well as to disseminate expertise.

Education and Training

Medical/nursing education is the ideal time to introduce the concept of deprescribing (alongside prescribing itself). The next generation of prescribers should be inspired to seek opportunities to identify and discover knowledge and expertise useful to this effort, hold their seniors to account on this burgeoning practice, and instigate innovation.

The current bias in class time towards initiating and continuing versus discontinuing medications is striking. Psychiatry residency programs should consider incorporating training in deprescribing into their core prescribing curricula. Knowledge, skills, and attitudes should be addressed in key competency areas such as (1) "What to prescribe"—psychopharmacology and critical appraisal of evidence; (2) "How to prescribe"—psychotherapeutically informed prescribing; and (3) "Why to prescribe"—ethical consideration, shared decision-making, and social justice. Each of these questions could then be asked again, with "deprescribing" as the subject.

The field of psychiatry should openly and nondefensively join productive public forums to consider and debate the potential benefits and risks of medications. The spirit of shared decision-making might also include voices from our field being heard in the wealth of consumer-driven public forums that exist online. Concerted public education, highlighting deprescribing as an area of interest and priority for psychiatry, may help reinforce the relevance and value of our field in these challenging times.

References

Alexander, L., & Druss, B. (2012). *Behavioral Health Homes for People with Mental Health and Substance Use Conditions: The Core Clinical Features.* Washington, DC: SAMHSA-HRSA Center for Integrated Health Solutions, US Department of Health and Human Services.

Coffin, W. S. (2004). *Credo.* Louisville, KY: Westminster John Knox Press.

Davies, J., & Read, J. (2018). A systematic review into the incidence, severity and duration of antidepressant withdrawal effects: Are guidelines evidence-based? *Journal of Addictive Behaviors*, doi.org/10.1016/j.addbeh.2018.08.027.

Deegan, P. E. (2004). Remember my name: Reflections on spirituality in individual and collective recovery. https://www.patdeegan.com/pat-deegan/lectures/remember-my-name

Gawande, A. (2009). *The Checklist Manifesto: How to Get Things Right.* New York: Henry Holt and Company.

Ostrow, L., Jessell, L., Hurd, M., Darrow, S. M., & Cohen, D. (2017). Discontinuing psychiatric medications: A survey of long-term users. *Psychiatric Services, 68*(12), 1232–1238.

Read, J., Cartwright, C., & Gibson, K. (2018). How many of 1829 antidepressant users report withdrawal effects or addiction? *International Journal of Mental Health Nursing, 27*(6), 1805–1815.

Steingard, S. (2018). Five year outcomes of tapering antipsychotic drug doses in a community mental health center. *Community Mental Health Journal, 54*(8), 1097–1100.

Stockmann, T., Odegbaro, D., Timimi, S., & Moncrieff, J. (2018). SSRI and SNRI withdrawal symptoms reported on an internet forum. *International Journal of Risk & Safety in Medicine*(Preprint), 1–6.

Weaver, M. (2018). Benzodiazepines. In T. S. Schepis, ed. *The Prescription Drug Abuse Epidemic: Incidence, Treatment, Prevention, and Policy* (pp. 47). Santa Barbara, CA: ABC-CLIO.

Appendix

Collaborative Deprescribing Worksheet (Part A)						
Reviewing what medications are you currently taking						
What?		How you take it? (directions)	Why do you take it? (original indication)	Current and potential . . .		Discuss ✓
Medication name	Dose/ form . . .			Pros	Cons	

Collaborative Deprescribing Worksheet (Part B)					
Deciding which medication to deprescribe					

What factors are most important to you in choosing? (e.g., number of pills, side effects, cost, preventing hospital admission)	What do you hope to happen? Anything you are concerned about?	Who should we involve in your deprescribing decision? (e.g., family, supports, providers)

What are the potential benefits and risks of deprescribing?

(You might want to discuss a few options before choosing one medication to deprescribe at this time)

Option 1		Option 2		Option 3	
Benefits	Risks	Benefits	Risks	Benefits	Risks

Medication to deprescribe:	

Collaborative Deprescribing Worksheet (Part C)			
Deprescribing plan			
Supports, Resources, and Wellness Strategies			
What to expect	What to try	Call me if . . .	Seek urgent care if . . .
Event Log			
Date /time	Proposed Action (med dose/ directions change, appointment or activity)	Any changes you noticed?	Anything you did in response?

Event Log continued			
Date /time	Proposed Action (med dose/ directions change, appointment or activity)	Any changes you noticed?	Anything you did in response?

Collaborative Deprescribing Worksheet Guidelines

- This document is designed to be completed and maintained by both the patient and prescriber as a framework to help guide, promote, and document a person-centered collaborative deprescribing process (it should not be overvalued as the core intervention in and of itself).
- There are three parts which can be used independently or together as one document: Part A documents information-gathering and sharing; Part B documents a shared decision-making process; and Part C documents details the implementation of the deprescribing plan (while allowing for flexibility).
- In Part A, gain a shared understanding of *all* current medications taken (this may include alternative remedies if relevant). Collaborate on listing both the current and potential future "pros versus cons" of taking each medication in commonly understood language. These may include pertinent positive and negative effects as well as other factors like cost and convenience that emerge from your discussion. Potential side effects should be curated to those most relevant (avoid simply listing all possible associated side effects of each medication). You should extend into further rows of the worksheet (and an additional Part A page) if needed. As you work through the worksheet, flag up to three medications that either the patient or the prescriber wishes to consider further for deprescribing. It is suggested that a prescriber and patient undertake Part A periodically, whether or not intending it to lead to a deprescribing. Part A refers to deprescribing Steps 1 through 4, detailed in Chapter 7.
- In Part B, the patient and prescriber, soliciting additional input as appropriate, engage in shared decision-making around which medication to deprescribe at this time. First, the patient identifies what factors/values are most important to him or her when making this decision (responding to the four direct questions). The patient's ideas, concerns, and expectations are elicited. The provider may assist the patient in identifying who else might be appropriate to involve in the deprescribing decision process—this may include key supports, peers, other providers, or consultants (such as pharmacists or other specialists). Once these foundations are in place, up to three medications (as identified in Part A) are examined in detail, asking the question: What are the potential benefits and risks of *deprescribing* the medication? Please note that, in contrast, in Part A, the pros and cons of *continuing* each medication are examined. In Part B, the prescriber and patient list the reasons for *discontinuing* the medication. Part B refers to deprescribing Steps 4 and 5 in Chapter 7.
- Part C—plan, do, study, act—refers to deprescribing Steps 6 and 7 in Chapter 7.
- At the end of each clinical encounter, the event log may be updated with agreed recommendations (and a copy made to chart).
- Each party is invited to sign their names to reflect the collaborative nature of the process.
- Consider adding a digital version of this document to your local health informatics systems.

Index

Page numbers followed by *b, f,* and *t* indicate boxes, figures, and tables, respectively.

For the benefit of digital users, indexed terms that span two pages (e.g., 52–53) may, on occasion, appear on only one of those pages.